THE WHITE PLAGUE

THE WHITE PLAGUE

Tuberculosis, Man, and Society

René *and* Jean Dubos

FOREWORD BY

David Mechanic

INTRODUCTORY ESSAY BY

Barbara Gutmann Rosenkrantz

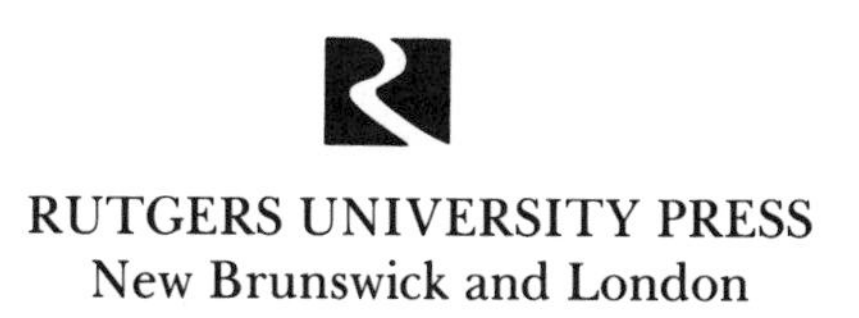

RUTGERS UNIVERSITY PRESS
New Brunswick and London

First published in 1952 simultaneously by Little, Brown and Company, Boston, and McClelland and Stewart Limited, Canada.

British Cataloguing-in-Publication information available.

Library of Congress Cataloging-in-Publication Data

Dubos, René J. (René Jules), 1901–
The white plague.

Bibliography: p.
Includes index.
1. Tuberculosis—History. 2. Tuberculosis—
Social aspects. I. Dubos, Jean, 1918–
II. Title. [DNLM: 1. Tuberculosis—popular works.
WF 200 D817w]
RC310.D82 1987 614.5'42'09 86-22033
ISBN 0-8135-1223-9
ISBN 0-8135-1224-7 (pbk.)

Manufactured in the United States of America

Contents

Foreword

THERE IS A LONG epidemiological tradition that examines the interrelations between disease agents, characteristics of the host, and the broader socio-cultural and environmental context. René Dubos, however, was unique in applying this perspective to a wide spectrum of issues ranging from microbiology to the quality of the environment. In his conception a combined epidemiological/ecological approach was not simply a methodological improvement in the understanding of health, but the basis of a humanistic philosophy that could help preserve the best qualities of mankind through the awareness of the complex interrelationships between populations and their environments.

During the nineteenth century, and throughout most of this one, tuberculosis was a widespread and deadly infectious disease. It was the source of a staggering amount of illness and mortality and engaged some of the best minds in the medical sciences. For many of these physicians tuberculosis was not only a scourge, but a disease they experienced personally either through their own illnesses or those of their loved ones. Like many writers, philosophers, and artists who took up tuberculosis as a theme, medical scientists developed a respect for the mystery of this disease, and its complex transactions with the environment.

Both authors of this classic volume, *The White Plague: Tuberculosis, Man, and Society*, had a personal as well as an intellectual involvement with tuberculosis. René Dubos's first wife died of the disease in 1942, and Jean Dubos, his co-author and second wife, had the disease as well. Their book reflects not only a broad knowledge and erudition in medical science and the humanities, but a deep intuitive understanding as well. It was an early exemplar of a now prevalent model for explicating the complex etiologic relations between agent, host, and environment, and an impressive analysis of how disease comes to be represented in public conceptions and how it serves as a metaphor for social ideologies. We have recently seen these themes brilliantly played out in Charles Rosenberg's *The Cholera Years* and Susan Sontag's perceptive essay *Illness as Metaphor. The White Plague* also serves as an instructive paradigm for such new threats as AIDS which fit more understandably within the analysis the Duboses present than within traditional biomedical conceptions. Like tuberculosis, AIDS is a social disease whose patterns of transmission must be understood not only through the activity of a microbe but equally through the study of attitudes, behavior, and social organization.

Dubos studied agricultural science in college in Paris, and between 1922 and 1924 was employed as the associate editor of the *Journal of International Agricultural Intelligence.* As an editor in Rome, he worked as a tourist guide to finance his passage to the United States. He met Dr. Selman Waksman while working in this capacity and, fortuitously, on his way to New York in 1924, encountered him again aboard ship. Waksman headed the soil microbiology division at the Agricultural Experiment Station at Rutgers University, and became Dubos's teacher when Dubos joined him there as a graduate student. Dubos received his Ph.D. from Rutgers in 1927 while working as a research assistant in soil microbiology and an instructor in bacteriology. His dissertation on the decomposition of cellulose by soil organisms living in varying environments reinforced an earlier realization that was to stay with him throughout his life—that organisms develop differently depending on environment, and that artificial, experimental conditions often fail to capture the richness of natural variability. This insight was not only a powerful tool in his study of health, disease, and human adaptation, but also subsequently made him a leader in developing a worldwide movement motivated by a respect for the complexity and beauty of ecological interconnections and concerned with the protection of the environment.

After receiving his Ph.D., Dubos joined the Department of Pathology and Bacteriology at the Rockefeller Institute for Medical Research, where he spent most of his career. In his early years he sought to learn how to decompose the envelope protecting the bacteria that caused lobar pneumonia. The search for an enzyme that could do the task led him to the study of swamp soil, and ultimately to the discovery of tyrothricin, a source of the first commercially produced antibiotics. Waksman, his mentor, later isolated streptomycin from soil microbes, a discovery that earned him the Nobel Prize, and resulted in the development of broad-spectrum tetracyclines.

Following two years as a professor at Harvard, Dubos returned to the Rockefeller Institute in 1944 and took up a project on the cultivation of tubercule bacilli where he made significant methodological advances that gave impetus to experimental research. Dubos became immersed in examining the occurrence of tuberculosis and susceptibility to it in the broadest sense. *The White Plague*, the compendium of his studies published in 1952, remains both illuminating and pleasurable to read some thirty-five years later.

The themes first developed in *The White Plague* were to define the scientific, environmental, and humanistic positions that were the mark of Dubos's enormous influence on the thinking of the educated public, as well as on scientists ranging in expertise from biology to sociology. As a prolific scholar, enthusiastic lecturer, and highly dedicated citizen Dubos repeatedly focused awareness on the degradation of the environment and stressed the need for ecological concerns. He thereby anticipated by decades current interests in the promotion of health and a safer environment by recommending a modification of how we live in and relate to the social world and to nature. While himself a dedicated medical scientist, he was critical of exaggerated claims about the effectiveness of solving health problems solely through medicine. He saw as a source of wonder the plasticity of living things—their own ability to develop structures and functions adaptive to local peculiarities. And he understood, and eloquently explained that "health and happiness cannot be absolute or permanent values, however careful the social and medical planning. Biological success in all its manifestations is a measure of fitness, and fitness requires never-ending efforts of adaptation to the total environment which is ever changing."

Adaptation was a key focus in Dubos's scientific thinking and philosophy. The problems of adaptation reflected the tensions between permanency and change, the past and the future. They also reflected the universal characteristics of man's nature, some dating back to our Paleolithic ancestors, others to the transient conditions of the moment, and still others to man's unique ability to set goals and follow a course of action. It was this ability to conceive a future, and to choose among alternatives in a social and ethical sense, that provided the crucial link between Dubos's scientific and humanistic perspectives.

It may seem curious than an eminent microbiologist who carried out so much of his scientific work on soils would have had such a large influence on the thinking of medical sociologists, ecologists, psychosocial epidemiologists, and environmentalists. Dubos himself explained his involvement with the social implications of adaptation. In *Man Adapting* he noted that his concern "with such problems emerged from an increasing awareness of the fact that the prevalence and severity of microbial diseases are conditioned more by the ways of life of the persons afflicted than by the virulence and other properties of the etiological agents."

Thus he believed that to make sense of the patterns of human disease required an understanding of man and his societies.

The approach Dubos encouraged has now become a prevalent model for the study of cardiovascular disease, cancer, mental illness, and most other chronic disease. The identification of social and personal risk factors, whether in the form of life-style, nutritional intake, or the orientation to work and social relationships, is today a common practice. The study of the complex interrelationships between social structure, psychological processes, and biology is itself now carried out under the rubric of a formal biopsychosocial model, an interdisciplinary paradigm increasingly useful to both investigators and clinicians. More research than ever before takes place at the boundaries of traditional disciplines, and the processes of interaction among systems constitute some of the most fascinating and challenging contemporary problems in the study of behavior.

René Dubos was a pioneer who introduced many of us to the marvels and significance of these transactions between man and environment and the extraordinary adaptiveness of organisms to changing conditions. However, as he knew, the human capacity to reconstruct the environment symbolically and to manipulate it physically opened new but sometimes threatening avenues. As both an outstanding scientist and a humanist of extraordinary breadth, he appreciated fully the havoc that man could bring upon himself. But he was also an optimist who believed that people of good will, harnessing their energies toward publicly constructive purposes, could contribute immeasurably to their own and others' well-being. Dubos was not only an analyst but an exemplar of the possibilities of human ingenuity.

David Mechanic, Ph.D.
René Dubos Professor of Behavioral Sciences
Rutgers University, New Brunswick
1987

Introductory Essay: Dubos and Tuberculosis, Master Teachers

Historians have been uncharacteristically reticent about disease and its influence on human life and society. The great plagues of antiquity and the middle ages were recorded by contemporaries, but few historians before the mid-twentieth century reckoned with the epidemics of modern times. Some scholars shied away because they felt ill-trained when it came to medical matters; others pointed to the paucity of sources. Yet all agreed that disease was a prevalent and destructive experience that threatened social order.

Tuberculosis provides a natural tutorial. Human history and the tubercle bacillus are so enmeshed that to follow the course of the disease over time is a prerequisite to understanding what the overall struggle to control disease means to ourselves and our contemporary society. Reading *The White Plague: Tuberculosis, Man, and Society*, a book that made such an understanding possible, led to reflections about the medical and social conception of tuberculosis that are explored in the three sections of this essay. The first concerns the shift of attention away from the sick person, and the presumption that everyone was susceptible to this common disease. After the discovery of the tubercle bacillus, in 1882, the significance of this new focus was particularly evident when the consumptive person came to be identified as the patient *with* tuberculosis—as someone who had contracted the disease through exposure to the microbe rather than through an inherent susceptibility. The second considers the ways that declining rates of death and disease from tuberculosis modified both scientific and popular beliefs about the underlying vulnerabilities to infection. The third examines some of the concerns about tuberculosis that surfaced after the introduction of antibiotics—once the control of contagion required less public vigilance and attention to personal hygiene.

It is over thirty years since René and Jean Dubos told the story of tuberculosis in *The White Plague*, a disease that now is as foreign to most young Americans as typhoid or diphtheria. Painful memories of tuberculosis have passed so far from public consciousness that *Newsweek* could recently run a story about Fred Schmidt, a sixty-nine-year-old man who survived a bout with the disease, as a human-interest feature. Schmidt recalled his own escape from the plague that killed his father and sister and the despair that came with the diagnosis. Tuberculosis once killed more people than any other single disease; the danger of death from consumption, as pulmonary tuberculosis was commonly called, tracked the footsteps of young men and women and loomed over courting couples for as long as they lived. Contracted in childhood or adolescence, tuberculosis left its victims more vulnerable to chronic or wasting illness in later years. In the middle of the nineteenth century diseases of the lung caused up to 25 percent of all deaths reported, and early in the twentieth century, when Americans were generally healthier, tuberculosis continued to head the list of fatal contagious diseases although it resulted in fewer deaths. Even when tuberculosis had slipped to seventh place in the roster of fatal diseases by 1930, it remained terribly destructive—the most frequent cause of death or disability during the critical ages of fifteen through forty-five.[1] During that time, the uncertainties of treatment also

1. In 1900, annual death rates from tuberculosis for white Americans were between 190 and 200 per 100,000. Among black Americans, however, the comparable figure was 400 deaths per 100,000, approxi-

magnified the public's fear of contagion. When a man was found to have tuberculosis he received a notice to quit his job and schoolchildren with the disease were ordered to stay home indefinitely. Thus, while most Americans today never have a brush with the disease, a bare half-century ago few children and adults were far from the experience or threat of tubercular infection.

Tuberculosis, however, was already a less ominous disease for the audience that read *The White Plague* when it was first published in 1952. By the mid-twentieth century—although close to 100,000 new cases of tuberculosis were reported each year—the annual number of deaths from the disease was declining rapidly from 34,000 to 11,000. Those dying were most likely to be the very old, or the malnourished and medically indigent—social outcasts or immigrants from remote nations where economic development had faltered. René and Jean Dubos called tuberculosis "a social disease" in order to associate the disease with poverty, although the term was more commonly associated with sexually transmitted diseases. Nonetheless, calling tuberculosis a social disease helped them make their point that although tuberculosis was contagious, more than simple contact with a tubercular person was necessary to become infected with it. Economic and social conditions, the Duboses stressed, were critical factors in its transmission. Moreover, they found that tuberculosis had profound social consequences in that it affected the "emotional and intellectual climate of the societies it attacked."[2] The enor-

mately the same level recorded in the middle of the nineteenth century for the population as a whole. In the United States, for the past fifty years, morbidity, rather than mortality, has been a better reflection of the danger of tuberculosis. Today, the tuberculosis death rate is less than 4 per 100,000 and the disease is even less visible than suggested by these figures since fatal disease occurs most often among the very old and debilitated.

2. René and Jean Dubos, *The White Plague: Tuberculosis, Man, and Society* (Boston, 1952; rpt. New Brunswick, N.J.: Rutgers University Press, 1987), vii.

mous burden of wasting illness and death caused by tuberculosis was interlocked with the industrial and urban transformations of the modern nation.

Therefore, although there is paleontological and textual evidence of tuberculosis early in human history, it is emphatically a disease of the nineteenth century, with social and medical symptoms that typify cultures in the midst of industrialization. *The White Plague* is a study of the changing values and symbols that came with the Industrial Revolution, and of the seemingly inexplicable, pervasive, and ravaging disease that appeared in tandem with it.

Alongside their account of the social ecology of tuberculosis, the Duboses celebrate the history of scientific research that culminated in Robert Koch's discovery of the tubercle bacillus in 1882. Koch's identification of the organism causing tuberculosis carried the work of many earlier investigators to a successful conclusion. Critical questions raised by previous observations were answered as a result of his laboratory breakthrough. It was at last possible to show the common pathology of different symptoms and the necessary bacterial origin of every tubercular infection.

These parallel histories, the first examining the complex social environment that generated the conditions of disease, and the second celebrating the growth of scientific knowledge about the biology of tuberculosis, added an important tension to the Duboses' narrative, a tension more apparent today than it may have been when the book was originally published. On the one hand, despite the terrible conditions found in the slums of industrial cities, the proportion of deaths from tuberculosis began to decline after the mid-nineteenth century. Resistance to infection was the best explanation for this fall in death rates. It was also the best hope for a further reduction in mortality since the conventional treatment of rest therapy was costly and other remedies were ineffective. On the other hand, the discovery of the tubercle bacillus and the demonstration of its necessary role in disease failed, at first, to change the minds of many doctors and of the public, who continued to blame the incidence of tuberculosis on heredity, climate, or psychogenic causes. Whatever the exact reason or prejudice, the idea of a single cause for a disease that affected the lives of so many people was not readily accepted.

But if the cause of tuberculosis is less debatable when *The White Plague* was first published, the menace of tuberculosis remained troublingly close during the 1940s. Despite effective measures to control the spread of infection, once the symptoms of tuberculosis became evident the disease was entrenched and resisted treatment. The new antibiotics could promise no cure when it came to tuberculosis. Earlier in the decade, Dr. Selman Waksman, Dubos's mentor, had isolated streptomycin, a powerful bacteriostatic that inhibited the growth of the tubercle bacillus. But within a short time the limitations of streptomycin in treating tuberculosis patients were known. Evidence that pathogenic organisms, including the tubercle bacillus, developed drug-resistant strains underscored the potential for medical disaster and the need for therapeutic prudence.

As René and Jean Dubos traced the history of tuberculosis in human societies, the events they examined moved closer and finally overtook their own personal and laboratory experiences; it became impossible to isolate the history of scientific knowledge from the history of the disease. Moreover, while researching the multiple historical configurations of tuberculosis, the Duboses found new meaning to their observation that "[N]ature reveals many roads that lead in the direction of truth."[3] Recognizing that the diminished threat of tuberculosis and the potential success of antibiotics could produce a therapeutic shortcut to disease control that might transform the human experience of ill-

3. Ibid., 70.

ness altogether, the Duboses nevertheless warned against the illusion of "conquering" disease. They perceived a danger in the scientific and social logic that aimed to treat the disease rather than to modify the underlying causes of vulnerability, and their own moral logic served to inform their history of tuberculosis.

I.

Contemporary medicine takes its lessons from observations of disease. Although the course of one patient's illness may differ from another's, each specific case is measured against a common standard developed out of a painstaking study of illness in many patients, from which the pathology of each particular disease has been generalized. For example, say Jane and John each has a case of measles. Their individual illnesses no longer inform our expectations about the course of their disease, because we know for certain that measles is a contagious disease commonly seen in children, marked by fever and a rash that starts at the head and upper body and gradually covers the child's trunk and extremities. After five or six days the rash fades, and gradually disappears; again, first from the head, shoulders, and upper trunk, and finally from the legs and feet. Early in the course of illness white patches, known as Koplik's spots, may be detected inside the cheek and on the roof of the mouth. A well-defined case ordinarily confers immunity and complications can be enumerated and described in the same way as a "normal" case of measles.

Tuberculosis presents more challenges given the multiplicity of its symptoms and their complex evolution; nonetheless, we expect a professional diagnosis to uncover the characteristic stigmata of the disease, and to predict its likely outcome. Not even a well-trained physician would diagnose tuberculosis without an

X-ray and other procedures, to distinguish between the coughs, sputum, and breath-sounds that different pulmonary diseases have in common, but the object of close scrutiny is more likely to be the disease rather than the patient. Excessive attention to individual differences among patients only complicates the task, even though these differences may alter the prognosis positively as well as negatively. In many ways we share the doctor's perspective. There is, after all, security in knowing that, no matter who the patient, measles will not turn into tuberculosis and that, with reasonable precautions, a grandfather's case of tuberculosis is not likely to appear in other members of the family.

These obvious and unquestionably useful assumptions about the cause and nature of illness guide us daily, but would have seemed ignorant and deceptive to the nineteenth-century physician, nurse, and public. Vulnerability to illness and fortitude in the face of disease were the underpinnings of an individual's fortune and fate; these aspects of character were determined by nature and manipulated by the wise physician in concert with the patient. Hence, the patient's constitution and temperament as well as circumstance were believed to impose a character upon the disease. Variations in sickness and death rates demonstrated differences among individuals and in the nineteenth century such idiocyncracies were used to identify and explain susceptibility to disease. As long as tuberculosis was prevalent at all ages the observed differences between individuals remained the accepted determinant of who would become ill. As a result, the combination of widespread lung disease and variable mortality rates stimulated studies of the patterns of mortality that would identify an individual's "tubercular diathesis," the name used to describe the characteristics of an individual's inherent vulnerability.

Nineteenth-century investigators such as Henry Ingersoll Bowditch concluded that the best way to avoid tuberculosis was to be born to parents who had not contracted the disease; the course of disease as well as its onset were predicted by circumstances of birth. Sex, occupation, the national origin of one's parents, and one's current residence were also considered important factors in determining whether one was likely to become tubercular.[4] While the debate over how tuberculosis was communicated raged on, the critical question of risk always centered on the constitution of the endangered individual.

The "golden age" of bacteriology challenged this view. Once the specific organism that produced a particular disease and its role in transmitting the disease from a sick to a healthy person was elucidated, the difference between being infected or free from infection became the only crucial distinction among individuals. Exactly how this principle of *equal* susceptibility came to be understood is, of course, what historical research can clarify. Applying the principle of *specific* contagion could also have led researchers to the conclusion that everyone was equally susceptible, but they often found it difficult to ignore evidence that certain parents and environments produced excessively large numbers of offspring who became tubercular, even when bacteriologists pointed out that these conditions could have generated tuberculosis only if the tubercle bacillus, the organism that actually caused the disease, was present.

The discovery and classification of many of the microscopic organisms that caused diphtheria, typhoid, erysipelas, and other prevalent diseases finally made it possible to understand and emphasize the *common* characteristics of susceptibility to infection in the absence of acquired immunity. Without an exposure to specific pathogens individual differences were of little consequence. Put another way, it became clear that a contagious disease could be controlled simply by restricting the activities and contacts of the person who was actually sick, since almost every-

4. Henry Ingersoll Bowditch, *Consumption in New England: or Locality One of Its Chief Causes* (Boston: Ticknor & Fields, 1862).

one else was susceptible. This underscored the effectiveness of quarantine, which was hardly a novel proposal. From our present perspective, it would seem that any new attempts to identify the conditions that made a sickness communicable should have appeared reasonable if they confirmed associations between personal behavior, social conditions, and the incidence of disease that were generally acknowledged from previous experience.

Yet, because tuberculosis was so common and so often chronic, there was a strong resistance to the proposed emphasis on the detection and control of infection rather than on the assessment of susceptibility and the manipulation of resistance to the disease. Frequently, physicians were alienated by the new vogue of investigation that focused on the bacteriological origins of tuberculosis and the predictable pathology of the disease. Doctors had been trained to notice the symptoms that called attention to differences among the sick. Medical care of tubercular patients traditionally took special account of personal habits and housing, and advice on how to live long and well despite a family history of tuberculosis was widely disseminated by physicians attending patients who were in a position to follow the latest instructions.

It was obvious, however, that the disease-oriented hygienic regimen dictated by bacteriological research came to grief when a patient's poverty made it unlikely that such advice would be followed. In the *Handbook for Practical Workers in the Tuberculosis Campaign* Ellen N. LaMotte identified the dilemma that the visiting nurse faced more dramatically than most physicians. Her book began with an instructive history: "The enormous prevalence of tuberculosis is due to the fact that its infectious nature was not recognized until 1882 when Koch discovered the bacilli." Since we now know that tuberculosis is a transmissable disease, she continued, we know it can be prevented through the exercise of proper precautions. But vigilance was not equally distributed. LaMotte assembled facts showing that tuberculosis was principally a disease of the poor, afflicting both those who were "financially handicapped and so unable to control their environment," and "those who are mentally and morally poor, and lack intelligence, will power, and self control." Her conclusion that "People of this sort . . . constitute almost the entire problem —otherwise the situation would be so simple that the word problem would not apply," conflicted uncomfortably with her intention of encouraging nurses to go forth and help the poor to defend themselves against tuberculosis. The reluctance of the poor to leave their homes for hospital care combined with the small number of beds in public hospitals for tuberculosis patients conspired to spread contagion. LaMotte repeatedly drew the picture of "a patient surrounded by a group of people able to offer but slight opposition to this insidious disease"—for example, a sick father lying in bed surrounded by his children, unwilling to "use his sputum cup, or take any other precautions—to illustrate, as she wrote, the "wrong conditions of relief-giving."[5]

Robert Koch himself had understood the massive obstacles to controlling "the disease of the masses." As soon as he reported his success in cultivating the tubercle bacillus, he was already considering the practical applications of his laboratory findings. In his opinion, the contagious nature of tuberculosis had been demonstrated earlier, and although the discovery of the bacillus strengthened arguments in favor of preventive measures, he knew that "owing to the great spread of this disease, all steps which are taken against the same will have to reckon with the social condition, and, therefore, it must be carefully considered in what way and how far one may go on this road without prejudicing the advantages gained, by unavoidable disturbances and

5. Ellen N. LaMotte, *The Tuberculosis Nurse: Her Functions and Qualifications: A Handbook for Practical Workers in the Tuberculosis Campaign* (New York: G. P. Putnam's Sons, 1915), 3, 4, 243, 231.

other disadvantages."[6] The prevalence of tuberculosis made it essential to note the personal and social characteristics of its victims that could guide selective intervention. Otherwise, general prophylaxis might be little more than propaganda—one contemporary called the educational films of the National Tuberculosis Association "crooked and unreal."[7] In the context of the NTA's warnings about the peril of exposure to widespread disease, this critic argued that only the callous would advise a regime of personal hygiene.

II.

A scientific perspective shapes the Duboses' history of tuberculosis. In the early twentieth century, medical researchers drew lessons from their observations of the reciprocity between parasite and host. Adopting an approach to the study of pathology that new research has continued to enhance, the Duboses showed how "to make sense" of nature, and thus how to place the history of disease in the service of the history of mankind. Since René Dubos elaborated the social implications of an underlying commensualism among living organisms in each of his popular books, it is not surprising that the natural and the social histories of tuberculosis became the fabric from which *The White Plague* was fashioned.

Dubos thereby joined a long and distinguished line of social commentators who saw in the patterns of mortality the interplay

6. Robert Koch, "Aetiology of Tuberculosis," translated by Rev. F. Sause, *American Veterinary Review* 13 (1889–1890): 214.
7. Randolph S. Bourne, "The Heart of the People," *The New Republic*, July 3, 1915: 233. Bourne condemns the National Tuberculosis Association educational film *The White Terror* as bad melodrama and cruel misrepresentation.

of natural and social forces. Throughout history, the seemingly self-evident connections between scientific knowledge and moral behavior have prevailed when it comes to explaining why some people were healthier than others. And, unquestionably, the laws of life that emerged from these scientific observations and became the basis for the control of disease were disputed as the historical context changed. Just a hundred years before *The White Plague* was published a doctor's popular text on the prevention of consumption opened a chapter on female health with traditional observations about preordained nature. "God is not unjust and partial," reflected Dr. Samuel Sheldon Fitch, "he has not made one to live one hundred and sixty years, while another cannot live more than twenty or thirty." From this truth the doctor deduced the conventional wisdom that women are themselves to blame for their premature deaths. To reinforce the point he later argued that the reciprocity of justice and pleasure means that "there is a high moral duty . . . the female owes [it] to her family, to her country, and the world . . . to preserve her charms—to keep the flowers of her own loveliness from fading."[8]

Tuberculosis did strike vulnerable individuals with extra vengeance, and the search for causal connections led investigators to identify characteristics and circumstances that seemed to suit the story and make hard facts more palatable to contemporaries. In the opera *La Boheme*, the heroine Mimi's death was cast in a romantic light, but more than sentiment brought Mimi to her deathbed, for it was well-known that young women succumbed to tuberculosis more often than young men. History regularly provided art and science with predictable instances of a woman's flawed condition. Before the Civil War, Dr. Josiah Curtis, a Massachusetts physician and statistician, pointed out that since males

8. Samuel Sheldon Fitch, *Six Discourses on the Functions of the Lungs; and Causes, Prevention, and Cure of Pulmonary Consumption, Asthma, and Diseases of the Heart* (New York: S. S. Fitch and Co., 1853), 190, 193.

were at a greater risk of death throughout their lives, the larger number of girls and women dying from tuberculosis restored the balance of nature. When it came to diagnosis, popular nineteenth-century lore held that women spat blood during menstruation, so that doctors might misconstrue the most reliable sign of tuberculosis. And in the twentieth century an authoritative medical text provided a chapter entitled the "Influence of Sex," considering several purported ramifications of tuberculosis, including the dangers presented by a woman's reproductive organs. Pointing out that tuberculosis often went into remission during pregnancy, but that the reverse was generally true after delivery, the author concluded, archly, that "[A]nalogous physiologic changes in males have not been associated with tuberculous infection."[9] Male/female differences in rates of tuberculosis continued to be observed, and as recently as 1952 a study of adolescents indicated that differences in nutritional status associated with hormonal changes at puberty might account for unequal sex ratios of tuberculosis.[10]

These and other suppositions about the epidemiology of tuberculosis created simplistic stereotypes, and vulgar explanations were dressed up to suit social conventions that went unquestioned. For instance, among blacks, mortality from tuberculosis was twice as high as for whites at the close of the nineteenth century, and that proportion continued when mortality rates declined as a whole. The author of a well-informed

9. Arnold Klebs, ed., *Tuberculosis: A Treatise by American Authors on its Etiology, Pathology, Frequency and Semiology, Diagnosis, Prognosis, Prevention, and Treatment* (New York: D. Appleton and Co., 1909), 83–84. The author of the chapter on diagnosis in *Tuberculosis* states, on page 214, that hemoptysis occurs in the "premenstrual period, during which there is a systemic plethora. . . ."

10. *Massachusetts Registry of Births, Marriages and Deaths*, Eighth and Tenth Annual Reports (1850 and 1851). Also see the *Index Medicus* (1951, 1952) under "tuberculosis" for articles citing the nitrogen and phosphorus retention and requirements for female adolescents.

and popular book, *Consumption, Its Relation to Man and His Civilization, Its Prevention and Cure*, published in 1906, was at great pains to eliminate what was called "phthisophobia," a mindless fear of infection. Uncertainties about the spread of the disease led employers to fire men with tuberculosis, forbade barbers in some towns from shaving consumptives, and authorized the U.S. Commissioner of Immigration to exclude foreigners with tubercular symptoms. The author poured out his indignation over this ignorance about the conditions in which tuberculosis might prove dangerous, but somehow the section of his book on "Races and Peoples" was left unaffected. After reporting that "the negro's small lung capacity, as compared with that of the white, and his deficient brain capacity render him less resistant to the disease when once acquired," he rested his case with the warning that "unless the hygienic and moral surroundings of the race are improved there is danger of its extinction."[11]

In these efforts to understand the pattern of unequal susceptibility to the disease, the unacknowledged social and personal values of the commentators appear to us as naively evident. Modern western cultures share the expectation that theory and facts will inform the practice of scientific medicine; in the cases cited above we can see, in retrospect, a blatant confounding of science with opinion. Without the use of historical lenses the diagnoses and prognoses of the past appear, at best, as foolish, at worst, as vicious. Contemporary accounts of the antecedents to poor health need to be assessed in the light of more recent knowledge. What historical demography actually bears out is that an exposure to a multiplicity of infectious diseases during the nineteenth century may well have compromised resistance to tuberculosis and prepared the way for later breakdowns under physical stress, such as childbirth. Thus, a recent detailed study of

11. John Bessner Huber, *Consumption, Its Relation to Man and His Civilization, Its Prevention and Cure* (Philadelphia: J. B. Lippincott Co., 1906), 445, 103.

deaths from epidemic diseases in Philadelphia at the turn of the century has opened the way for a reconsideration of a late nineteenth-century scientific thesis that pointed to an apparent connection between lowered typhoid mortality and other contagious diseases.[12] However, in general, nineteenth-century scientists noted predispositions to consumption that made moral sense of nature's ways. Connections that they saw between dirt and disease, between social norms and biological "facts," are connections that we have partly refuted. As a result it often seems as though the patterns of susceptibility reported a century ago were peculiarly judgmental in comparison to our more liberal social calculus.

It was when common knowledge mirrored science, as in the assumption that acquired immunity after infection provided protection against future disease, that medical practice began to distance itself from moral values. As twentieth-century epidemiologists examined the changing age distribution of tuberculosis mortality and began to untangle the critical relationship between early infection and later disease, it gradually became evident that when tuberculosis mortality decreased there would be complementary alterations in the pattern of disease. During the 1930s, Wade Hampton Frost, a doctor who set the guidelines for the discipline of epidemiology in the U.S. Public Health Service, tried out different theories to explain the changing picture of susceptibility and resistance to tuberculosis. With each succeeding generation tuberculosis seemed to strike at an older age, an observation that at first suggested that early tuberculosis infection gave temporary protection, and the price of health in child-

12. William T. Sedgwick and J. Scott MacNutt, "On the Mills Reincke Phenomenon and Hazen's Theorem Concerning the Decrease in Mortality From Diseases Other than Typhoid Fever Following the Purification of Public Water Supplies," *Journal of Infectious Diseases* 7 (1910):489–564; Gretchen A. Condran and Rose A. Cheney, "Mortality Trends in Philadelphia: Age- and Cause-Specific Death Rates 1870–1930," *Demography* 19 (February 1982):97–123.

hood was disease in later life when vigor waned. This new definition of risk (that once would have been called predisposition), together with the recognition that reduced rates of tuberculosis were largely the result of a general improvement in health and living conditions, began to affect established stereotypes about the disease. In a significant way, as the Duboses pointed out two decades later, it became both possible and necessary for researchers to take into account the role of social factors while working out the epidemiology of tuberculosis.

Public health policy and practice were influenced by this modified perspective about the dangers of the tubercle bacillus. When tuberculosis sanatoria had opened during the last decades of the nineteenth century, early treatment was considered the best assurance of recovery, which led to the preferential admission of patients whose disease was not far advanced, and those at special risk because poverty had left them ill-equipped to care for themselves. It was believed that, with modest precautions, tuberculosis was not highly contagious except in the last stages of "open" disease. Therefore, those patients with advanced cases of tuberculosis were cared for only when limited medical services became available. In the middle of the Great Depression Dr. Frost considered this program of treatment with misgivings: "How far the tuberculosis control program should extend in the direction of general social betterment is a question which," he wrote, "perhaps need not be answered." As his understanding of tuberculosis epidemiology developed he recognized that "obviously, the tuberculosis control program cannot expand to include the whole scheme of social betterment," and began to advocate a future policy: "[T]he soundest principle [is] . . . that as the cases become fewer and fewer, preventive measures should be centered more and more upon open cases." At this dreadful time of massive unemployment it was particularly difficult to consider withdrawing general preventive assistance from the young and the poor who had historically been considered most at risk.[13]

Very shortly after the Depression new studies showed the need to modify the notion that immunity stemmed from a benign tuberculosis infection early in life. It became clear that many of the active cases of tuberculosis diagnosed in older adults were the result of a childhood infection. In an article published posthumously Frost wrote, "to have passed through a period of high mortality risk confers not protection, but added hazard in later life."[14] Between the two world wars, as new concepts of risk were adopted by epidemiologists studying contagious and "chronic" diseases, tuberculosis emerged more clearly again as a *social* disease. And not surprisingly, as the complex interactions between social and biological factors were better understood, the hope of assured protection from infection became, in some important respects, more remote. The search for an effective treatment, therefore, began to move away from prophylaxis toward active therapy, an avenue previously explored in the nineteenth century with tuberculin injection.

III.

What Changes has the Acceptance of the Germ Theory Made in Measures for the Prevention and Treatment of Consumption? was the title

13. Wade Hampton Frost, "How Much Control of Tuberculosis?" *American Journal of Public Health* 27 (1937):765, 766.

14. Wade Hampton Frost, "The Age Selection of Mortality from Tuberculosis in Successive Decades," *American Journal of Hygiene* 30 (1939):91–96. See also George W. Comstock, "Frost Revisited: The Modern Epidemiology of Tuberculosis," *American Journal of Epidemiology* 101 (1975):363–382. The Duboses point out that statistics from the Children's Chest Clinic of Bellevue Hospital indicate that recurrent disease in adolescents showed the earlier pattern of disproportionate female susceptibility; see *The White Plague*, 125–126.

of a report written by the Superintendent of the Providence, Rhode Island Health Department in 1888. Responding to his own question, Dr. Charles V. Chapin asserted that "there is no theoretical reason why a purely contagious disease like tuberculosis cannot be exterminated," though the prospects for treatment once the disease was established were less favorable. Chapin reached this guarded conclusion after reviewing two approaches to treatment; the first was designed to strengthen "bodily" resistance to tuberculosis through "climatic or hygienic treatment." Although prophylactic measures enjoyed a certain vogue, Chapin charged that they lacked scientific support and were founded on a "rational empiricism" that "owes little or nothing to the modern views of tubercular etiology." The alternative, he held, was a "medicinal treatment . . . offering the greatest attraction to the experimental and ambitious therapeutist[:] the application of germicidal agents to the pulmonary tissue." Yet, when Chapin reviewed various germicidal agents he concluded that despite the attraction of eradicating tuberculosis on the spot, there was no antiseptic that would do the job without serious injury to the patient. The sad truth was that, for the moment, germ theory advanced neither the hygienic nor the therapeutic controls of tuberculosis.[15]

Chapin's frustration strikes a note that is heard again today. Despite remarkable therapeutic accomplishments, we know that cures can themselves be hazardous. Microbial pathogens acquire "resistance" to treatment and stand as symbols of hubris in man's battle with nature; Dubos had examined this danger with respect to the use of streptomycin to treat tuberculosis. Other microorganisms—gonococci, staphlococci, and streptococci—continue to make news in the science columns of the daily pa-

15. Charles V. Chapin, *What Changes has the Acceptance of the Germ Theory Made in Measures for the Prevention and Treatment of Consumption?* Fiske Fund Prize Dissertation No. 38 (Providence: Providence Press Company, 1888), 44, 12.

pers because of variant strains that become dangerous after repeated exposure to antibiotics.

Chapin raised another theme that is familiar today. In principle, he argued, mankind can prudently control contagious disease by blocking the routes of transmission. Where the "fastidious" tubercle bacillus was concerned, survival of the organism depended on quite specific conditions; yet despite these potentially limiting requirements the disease was widespread. For Chapin, education was the solution to this apparent paradox. Doctors would have to undertake this task, since the public persistently resisted the measures that were required for the effective control of contagion. But there were differences of opinion on the choice of strategies among scientists as well; Robert Koch had earlier already been considerably less optimistic about the potential effectiveness of preventive measures. General prevention may well have been the best way around the dilemma of treatment, but the barriers to prevention seemed formidable, particularly to Koch, who had personally reckoned with the impediments of the German Imperial bureaucracy.

Under these conditions, Koch made his own significant contribution to the parade of therapies that had begun long before his 1882 discovery of the tubercle bacillus. His subsequent announcement of a "tuberculin" treatment in 1890, which gave little information about the agent itself, evoked predictable enthusiasm that continued even after strong evidence that patients often became sicker following the tuberculin injection. Americans were particularly unwilling to give up hope, and after tuberculin was discredited as a therapy, new cures often took desperate forms. No program of prevention or promising treatment was undertaken with full confidence of success, and every intervention demanded personal fortitude and social commitments that often exceeded whatever resources were available.

It almost seemed as if tuberculosis had been specially created to test national and personal character and to teach lessons of enduring significance. Indeed, the prospect of a cure itself evoked fears that if tuberculosis disappeared, other dangers might be unleashed; it was thought that this dread disease might block other unimaginable, festering plagues, that were beyond all prevention or remedy. Koch was not the only one who pointed out that tuberculosis was the visible symbol to contemporary social problems and inequities that resisted remedy.

Within the framework of ninteenth-century medicine it was taken for granted that tuberculosis was the manifestation of each victim's family heritage and personal history. However, in the light of twentieth-century scientific medicine information was acquired more directly; a X-ray and a positive response to tuberculin definitively indicated the presence of disease. It was, therefore, only in the realm of treatment that scientific medicine failed to clear the way for a direct assault on tuberculosis. Here the debates and disappointments continued and the contradictions were focused, even if there were genuine achievements such as the development of a protective vaccine by Albert Calmette and Alphonse Guerin. Bacillus Calmette Guerin (BCG) was introduced in France in the 1920s and widely adopted elsewhere although it was only effective *prior* to direct infection. In the United States BCG was greeted with mixed feelings, in part because in the process of stimulating immunity BCG induced a positive tuberculin reaction and thus eliminated the usefulness of this reaction in the detection of asymptomatic disease. Americans found it hard to accept a strategy that, in effect, could mask a true case of tuberculosis. Underlying assumptions about the determinants of susceptibility to tuberculosis were now, as always, critical to medical and public health practices, and calibrating risks and benefits necessarily depended on an amalgam of knowledge derived from different kinds of evidence. Yet, in the case of BCG it is hard not to speculate that its tepid reception by the American medical community was associated with the restrictive immigration policies of the 1920s and the related suspicion that immunization might hide otherwise detectable diseases.

The vision of conquering disease through scientific intervention has prompted hopes and fears: is it possible to eradicate tuberculosis and ignore the social pathology that produced susceptibility? René Dubos was affronted by utopian prophecies about a medical practice capable of creating a life free of disease and appalled at the corresponding neglect of disease-generating conditions. He knew how persistently false expectations were raised through science about the total eradication of disease. Even when he wished, as he did in 1952, that a new drug—isonicotinic acid hydrazide (isoniazid or INH) —would make his skepticism "obsolete," he warned that "Tuberculosis will be conquered only when man has learned to function according to a physiological way of living that renders him more resistant to tubercle bacilli, and when he has created a social environment that protects him from exposure to infection." Thirty years later, when writing an introduction to the Japanese translation of *The White Plague*, he reminded a new audience that although tuberculosis was now medically controlled in prosperous industrial nations, the underlying biological and social realities that produced both resistant organisms and poverty still persisted. Dubos observed that in New York City, where he lived, present-day victims of tuberculosis were likely to be immigrants from Puerto Rico and Haiti who were infected with tubercle bacilli that had acquired resistance to isoniazid and other chemotherapies, "a consequence of poor medical practices in the use of these drugs." Dubos turned to his knowledge of history to underscore the dangers of treating the symptoms of pathology—that is disease—and ignoring the "social factors" that produced susceptibility.[16]

16. *The White Plague*, p. 156. Japanese translation of *The White Plague* done for Japan Anti-Tuberculosis Society, 1982.

Tragedy masquerades as irony in this instance since society determined both the risks characteristic of tuberculosis victims and the anxieties of those who analyzed and explained these risks. As a scientist and a citizen of the world, Dubos was deeply conscious of the dangers inherent in the false illusions of security promoted by treating symptoms rather than the underlying disturbance. Like Ellen LaMotte, who feared the short-term solution, Dubos's confidence in the possibility of essential social betterment left him willing to forgo relief if it compromised long-term goals. Without minimizing the dangers of treatment that obscure the causes of disease, it is useful to remember that a "social disease" typically affects the socially marginal, who can ill-afford to wait for the fundamental insights and social transformations that challenge well-established associations of disadvantage and disease.

There are, of course, economic, political, and moral hazards to prevention as well, that we can perceive more clearly when the advantaged are at risk; the swine flu immunization program of 1976 is a case in point. A historical transformation of epidemiology has taken place in our own time now that tuberculosis is in principle, at least, "conquered"—in part by treatment—and the social disease of the moment is AIDS. Society may choose to prevent this disease rather than to treat it, but individuals themselves rarely have that choice.

Barbara Gutmann Rosenkrantz
Harvard University
Cambridge
1987

To Our Sources

Do not take offense at not finding your name in this book. We borrowed facts, ideas, and expressions from so many that it would have been impossible to give credit to all, and unfair to mention only a few. With Montaigne we should like to say:

> As by some might be saide of me: that here I have but gathered a nosegay of strange floures, and have put nothing of mine unto it, but the thred to binde them. Certes, I have given unto publike opinion, that these borrowed ornaments accompany me; but I meane not they should cover or hide me; it is contrary to mine intention, who would make shew of nothing that is not mine owne, yea mine owne by nature; and had I believed my selfe, at all adventure I had spoken alone.

Introduction to the First Edition

FROM THREE TO FIVE MILLION persons die of tuberculosis every year throughout the world. Some fifty million suffer from the disease and transmit the germ of infection to their fellow men. Yet in every continent, under every climate, and among men of every race, there are communities where tuberculosis is either completely absent or of little consequence; in fact, the disease has been practically wiped out from a few localities where it was once prevalent. Clearly, then, its destructive power is not the inevitable expression of geographic, climatic or racial factors. Men living in complex and industrialized societies can be as free of tuberculosis as once were the Indians, the Polynesians and the Eskimos before the white invader came to disturb their ancestral way of life.

Tuberculosis is a social disease, and presents problems that transcend the conventional medical approach. On the one hand, its understanding demands that the impact of social and economic factors on the individual be considered as much as the mechanisms by which tubercle bacilli cause damage to the human body. On the other hand, the disease modifies in a peculiar manner the emotional and intellectual climate of the societies that it attacks. It is this subtle interplay between the social body and the social disease which constitutes the central theme of the present study.

Information concerning any given disease is usually derived from mortality statistics, hospital records and medical writings.

But these documents are always incomplete, while inaccuracies of diagnosis and certain social conventions and taboos often distort the information that they pretend to convey. For this reason, we have made much use of another kind of knowledge, less precise in appearance than official and scientific statements, but at times more revealing and more trustworthy. Details of great medical interest are found in the letters, diaries and biographies, in the novels, plays and works of arts, by which men and women have attempted to describe their experience and their times. Thus, the ubiquitous presence of tuberculosis can be detected readily throughout the annals of the Western world in the nineteenth century. A great outburst of the disease followed the Industrial Revolution. The epidemic became the White Plague, giving pallor to the dreariness of the mushrooming cities, and injecting its fever into the romantic moods of the age.

The records of this not too distant and therefore comprehensible past will help us to become familiar with the disease through our senses and emotions; we shall become aware of its physical and psychic effects, of its influence on behavior and tastes. Then, we shall consider how understanding of the tuberculous process and mastery of preventive and therapeutic procedures have progressively developed from empirical observations and from scientific analysis. Finally, we shall attempt to synthesize from historical documents and from the facts revealed by scientific inquiry, a picture of the evolution of tuberculosis and of the manner in which society can overcome infection.

There will emerge from this synthesis the conclusion that tuberculosis is not, as Dickens believed, a disease that "medicine never cured, wealth never warded off." It is the consequence of gross defects in social organization, and of errors in individual behavior. Man can eradicate it without vaccines and without drugs by integrating biological wisdom into social technology, into the management of everyday life.

René and Jean Dubos

Part One

THE WHITE PLAGUE IN THE NINETEENTH CENTURY

CHAPTER I

The Captain of All the Men of Death

Diseases manifest multiple personalities just as do living creatures and social institutions. The various moods which they display in different circumstances and at any given time reflect the dominant aspect of the relationship between the disease process and the life of man in society.

Tuberculous infections have been described under many peculiar names in the course of history, and the meaning of old names has undergone great alteration with time. These changes are not due to whims or carelessness of thought, but to the fact that succeeding ages have looked at tuberculosis from various points of view, emphasizing different aspects of it. The never-ending metamorphosis of words is the method by which language adapts itself to the impact of new discoveries, and to changes in attitude concerning the nature of disease and its effect on man.

The expressions "lunger" of American slang and *poitrinaire* of French literature epitomize a type of patient suffering from a chronic, debilitating disease of the lungs, requiring at least several months, and usually many years, to run its course. This is the form of tuberculosis most commonly recognized in our society. But the disease can affect many organs other than the lungs. Thus, severe pulmonary tuberculosis is often accompanied by the production of lesions in the larynx and in the intestines; laryngeal tuberculosis renders swallowing extremely painful and can bring about an almost complete extinction of the voice; intestinal tuberculosis causes an exhausting diarrhea.

Involvement of certain lymphatic nodes is one of the constant manifestations of tuberculosis. The expressions "scrofulous" and "strumous glands" were frequently used in the past to describe these tuberculous nodes, particularly those of the neck. The adjective "scrofulous" suggests resemblance to a sow, and "strumous" means "something built up." Tubercle bacilli can become widely distributed throughout the body by way of the blood stream, causing a generalized infection called "miliary tuberculosis," which is characterized by the formation of very small nodules in most organs. Instead of becoming generalized, the disease can be limited to certain parts of the body. Inflammation of the membranes surrounding the brain (meningeal tuberculosis), destruction of kidney tissue (renal tuberculosis), the infirmity of the hunchback known as gibbus or Pott's disease (tuberculosis of the spine), lupus (tuberculosis of the skin), fistula-in-ano and several other pathological conditions illustrate the power of tubercle bacilli to cause destructive lesions in practically all tissues and organs. Indeed, the bacilli can also be the cause of infections that remain undiagnosed because of their atypical character — often so unspecific as to be dismissed under the name of cold or grippe, now and then acute enough to cause symptoms that are confused with typhoid-like fevers.

Tuberculosis can affect its victims in many different ways even when it remains chiefly localized in the lung. It may run a fulminating course, and bring about extensive destruction of lung tissue in a few months; this is the "galloping consumption" so often spoken of with terror in bygone days. Usually, however, it waxes and wanes with long periods of apparent remission followed by periods of exacerbation. Very often it is mistaken for a mild, chronic bronchitis, which allows the patient a normal span of life — in the course of which he harbors virulent bacilli and acts as a source of infection for his fellow men.

* * *

In the preceding paragraphs we have used the generic name "tuberculosis" for a whole group of diseases caused by tubercle bacilli. The word is so well-known today as to need no explanation, and yet it seems to have appeared in print for the first time around 1840, and has come into common use only during the past fifty years. Although the word is of such recent origin, it is probable that the disease itself is as old as mankind. Evidence of it has been found in a neolithic burial ground near Heidelberg, which has yielded the skeleton of a young man showing fusion of the fourth and fifth dorsal vertebrae. Thus, tuberculosis of the spine was already afflicting prehistoric man some six thousand years ago. Bone lesions probably caused by tubercle bacilli have also been recognized, both macroscopically and microscopically, in the mummified body of the venerable priest of Ammon, exhumed from a tomb of the Twenty-first Egyptian Dynasty, 1000 B.C. Indeed, other excavations in the same area have unearthed so many bodies with tuberculous lesions that the existence of a large sanatorium in ancient Egypt has been postulated. Many specimens of ancient drawings, potteries and statuary, obtained from many parts of the world, represent human beings with physical deformities characteristic of tuberculosis, thus providing further evidence that tubercle bacilli have long been the cause of human disease.

Descriptions that fit well the symptoms of pulmonary tuberculosis occur in the legends of many primitive people; in the early Hindu writings the disease is referred to by a word meaning "a consumption."[1] Translations of this word, for example, the Greek *phthisis,* seem to have been adopted in most ancient and modern languages to designate tuberculosis. But despite the recurrence of its name, it is not easy to evaluate the prevalence of the disease from a study of written documents.

Until late in the nineteenth century, many wasting diseases of the chest – cancer, silicosis, various lung abscesses – were confused with tuberculosis, even by the most experienced clinicians.[2]

On the other hand, it is only during modern times that certain types of nonpulmonary diseases have been recognized as being caused by tubercle bacilli and therefore belonging to the class of tuberculosis. As a consequence of these uncertainties of diagnosis, much of what is described as "consumption" in old medical writings was not really tuberculosis, whereas much actual tuberculosis remained unrecognized.

Moreover, many prejudices and practical reasons were responsible for keeping tuberculosis off the death records. The occurrence of a tuberculous death in a family was considered as a stigma, the disease being associated in the minds of most people with some obscure hereditary defect or with poverty. It decreased eligibility for marriage, for certain occupations and even for life insurance in other members of the family.

For all these reasons, it is impossible to obtain accurate data concerning the prevalence of tuberculous infection even during recent times. Nevertheless, its general trends can be recognized more readily than is the case with most other diseases, since many of the symptoms and pathological lesions of advanced "phthisis" are so characteristic as to be readily identified. Wasting fever, night sweats, breathlessness, pain in the side or shoulder, cough, abundance of sputum, and blood spitting have been associated with pulmonary consumption from the earliest times. Tubercles, cavities, and other typical lesions have been the telltale trace of the disease wherever autopsies have been performed. The frequency with which all these obvious manifestations are discussed by physicians and nonmedical writers gives some general indication of the relative importance of the disease at different times and in different civilizations. Its signs are described frequently and at length by Hindu, Greek and Roman writers, who lived in urban societies, but they are barely mentioned in the Bible and in other lore of pastoral peoples.

Another clue to the prevalence of tuberculosis in different periods of European history is found in the accounts of the ceremony of the "touch" performed by the French and English monarchs to cure the swollen glands that occur in the necks of those suffering from scrofula. Ever since Clovis in the fifth century, the kings of France were believed to receive from God this healing power at the time of their anointment; Edward the Confessor in the eleventh century had also claimed it for the English kings, and the Office remained in the Prayer Book until 1719. (Hence, the expression "king's evil," under which scrofula came to be known.) In *Macbeth,* Shakespeare describes how the king "touched" the scrofulous patients:

> . . . strangely-visited people
> All swol'n and ulcerous, pitiful to the eye,
> The mere despair of surgery, he cures,
> Hanging a golden stamp about their necks,
> Put on with holy prayers; and 'tis spoken,
> To the succeeding royalty he leaves
> The healing benediction . . .

Royal records reveal that on both sides of the Channel many thousands of pilgrims traveled yearly to be touched and cured by the king. The first act of Henry of Navarre, when he entered Paris as Henry IV in 1594, was to touch six hundred scrofulous persons.

In Rheims, the city where the French kings were anointed, a devout woman established in 1645 the Saint Marcoul Hospital for the care and isolation of the scrofulous patients who had traveled from far distances to be touched and had not been cured. Obviously, faith in the royal gift of healing, and life in the open air during the long trips to Rheims, did not always have the expected therapeutic effects. To express his skepticism, Rabelais wrote in *Pantagruel* of a queen who, outdoing the healing of scrofula by the touch, could cure all sorts of distemper with a song! But nevertheless, the practice continued in England and France until the end of the eighteenth century. According to Boswell, Samuel Johnson was one of the scrofulous to be touched in 1712 by Queen Anne, but he was not cured. The practice seems to have reached a maximum of popularity some time during the seventeenth century—a period when hospital records show that deaths from pulmonary consumption were particularly common in Europe. In England, the largest number of persons applying to be touched was recorded in 1684, when many of them were trampled to death in attempting to reach the hand of the king.

Definite statements concerning the frequency of the various groups of diseases in general medical practice and in large hospitals began to appear during the seventeenth century. They indicate that, although pulmonary phthisis was still rare in the country districts around 1650, it caused some 20 per cent of all deaths in England and Wales. It was a few decades later that John Bunyan wrote in *The Life and Death of Mr. Badman:* "The captain of all these men of death that came against him to take him away, was the Consumption, for it was that that brought him down to the grave." There are indications that tuberculosis mortality slowly decreased during the latter part of the seventeenth century, accounting for only 13 per cent of the deaths in 1715.[3] It began to increase again around 1730, and reached a maximum in England and America at the end of the eighteenth and during the first half of the nineteenth century. Witness to this fact is the testimony of many contemporary observers.

Returning from a survey of hospitals in Italy, the English physician, Benjamin Pugh, reported in 1784 that he had found in Rome "fevers of every class, but scarcely one where the lungs had not been primarily concerned." In France Antoine Portal wrote at the beginning of the nineteenth century, "There is no more dangerous disease than pulmonary phthisis, and no other is so common . . . it destroys a very great part of the human race." In England both Thomas Beddoes, in 1799, and William Heberden, in 1802, stated that pulmonary consumption was by far the most deadly disease. This opinion was echoed by Thomas

Young in an extensive review of all the important writings on phthisis published in 1815 in London under the title *Historical and Practical Treatise on Consumptive Diseases.* Said he, "Of all hectic affections, by far the most important is pulmonary consumption, a disease so frequent as to carry off prematurely about one-fourth part of the inhabitants of Europe, and so fatal as often to deter the practitioner even from attempting a cure." The situation was no better in the Eastern cities of the United States, where the annual tuberculosis mortality rate was of the order of 400 per 100,000 population. In the penitentiaries of Auburn, Boston and Philadelphia, 10, 11 and 13 per cent respectively of the white inmates died from phthisis between 1829 and 1845. The proportion was even higher among the Negro prisoners.

The bearing of these statements on the actual prevalence and mortality of tuberculosis is somewhat uncertain. Diagnosis being then based exclusively on signs and symptoms, the words "pulmonary consumption" and "phthisis" were often used to designate a variety of unrelated diseases. More reliable information is provided by the reports of those clinicians who attempted to determine the cause of death by conducting autopsies on their patients. The detailed accounts published by the French physicians of the early nineteenth century are particularly useful in this regard. Out of 696 autopsies performed at the Hôpital de la Charité in Paris by Gaspard L. Bayle in the early 1800's, there are some 250 cases in which death was almost certainly due to tuberculosis. The same proportion holds true in the series studied by René Théophile Laënnec a few years later.

The information concerning the prevalence of scrofula in the nineteenth century is particularly striking.[4] Approximately half of the English population had the disease. In 1844, all 78 boys and 91 of the 94 girls in a workhouse in Kent were found to be suffering from it, although only a few of them had shown obvious signs before being admitted to the institution. Similarly, 53 per cent of the children in a Berlin orphanage were found to be scrofulous. In the French Army, the mean rate of sickness from scrofula was of the order of 17 per 1000 in 1850. It is among the children brought from the East and West Indies and from the South Sea Islands to be educated in England that tuberculosis of the joints and glands seems to have caused the greatest ravages. "It is remarkable," states the *Lancet* of 1824, "that boys brought from tropical climates from the age of eight to twelve almost uniformly become scrofulous. They bear the first winter tolerably well, but droop during the second, and the third generally proves fatal to them." [5]

Tuberculosis was then unquestionably the greatest single cause of disease and death in the Western world, and one finds it masquerading throughout medical and nonmedical writings under a bewildering variety of names. Besides the words "phthisis," "consumption" and "scrofula," the expressions "asthenia," "tabes," "bronchitis," "inflammation of the lungs," "hectic fever," "gastric fever," "lupus," and many more, referred in most cases to conditions now known to have been caused by tubercle bacilli. The disease struck hardest among young men and women in their prime, condemning many of them to early death.

> Youth grows pale, and spectre thin, and dies,

wrote Keats in the spring of 1819.

It was probably to soften the sharp edge of the tragedy of premature death that the sinking of tuberculous youth was referred to as "going into a decline." But as the number of deaths mounted throughout the first half of the century, it became obvious that the gravity of the disease could no longer be concealed under genteel but misleading expressions. Tuberculosis was "The Great White Plague," threatening the very survival of the European race.

CHAPTER II

Death Warrant for Keats

ALL THE TRAGEDY of consumption, the perverted attitude of the romantic era toward the disease, and the ignorance of nineteenth century medicine concerning its diagnosis, nature and treatment are exemplified in the story of John Keats, dead tuberculous in 1821 at the age of twenty-six.[1]

Keats, the eternally young, is remembered more for his tragic death than for his vigorous enjoyment of life. The romanticized portrait transmitted to us by his contemporaries is that of the fragile poet who fell victim to tuberculosis because his sensitive nature had been unable to withstand contact with a crude world. It was through the mistaken idea that his disease had been precipitated by the brutal attack published against his poetry in the *Quarterly Review*, that Shelley symbolized him as Adonais — the youth who was mortally wounded by a wild boar and changed by Venus into an anemone. "The savage criticism on his *Endymion*," wrote Shelley in the introduction to *Adonais*, "produced the most violent effect on his susceptible mind. The agitation thus originated ended in the rupture of a blood vessel in the lungs; a rapid consumption ensued." But in reality, Keats was not unduly susceptible to critical opinion. He was not the frail flower so appealing to nineteenth-century tastes. He contracted tuberculosis because he was heavily exposed to infection and rendered more susceptible to it through unfortunate circumstances of life. The fatal issue of his disease was rendered almost inevitable by delayed diagnosis and by medical mismanagement.

As a boy, Keats first won recognition from his schoolmates, not as a scholar or a poet, but as a "bruiser," whose intensity of life found expression in boxing. The happiness of his school days was dispelled by the illness of his mother, who was suffering from an undiagnosed wasting disease. In 1809 the fourteen-year-old boy devoted his Christmas holidays to caring for her, allowing no one else to cook her food, or to give her medicine, and often sitting by her the entire night. Three months later Mrs. Keats died, "taken in a consumption."

Keats's acquaintance with disease and death was extended during the four years that he served as apprentice to an apothecary surgeon in Edmonton and later while he was a medical student at Guy's Hospital in London.[2] Although he did fairly well during his medical studies, and completed the course, poetry had taken control of his mind, and he soon realized that he was not interested in medicine. "There came a sunbeam into the room, and with it a whole troop of creatures floating in the ray," and there he was "off with them to Oberon and fairyland." He longed for the moments that he could snatch from class work to satisfy his craving for walks in the open country and identification with nature. One evening he read the newly published translation of Homer by Chapman, and within a few hours completed his first major poem, "On First Looking into Chapman's Homer." He could no longer escape the compulsion of his genius. The "bright star" had bewitched him, and he felt

> . . . like some watcher of the skies
> When a new planet swims into his ken . . .

The Keats brothers were in serious financial straits upon the completion of John's medical studies, and George, the eldest, left England to seek his fortune in the United States. Tom, the youngest, had been phthisical for several years and at the age of eighteen was ordered to South Devon in the hope that the mild climate might perform a cure. John spent two months with him there, during which time the brothers were confined to their room by almost constant rain. Tom was restless and, since his health did not improve, the brothers returned to London. Shortly after, John decided to accompany his friend, Armitage Brown, on a walking trip through Scotland and the Lake Country, obeying what was probably a subconscious urge to escape association with Tom's disease. The two friends walked for six weeks, averaging twenty miles a day through difficult country in bad weather, and often with little to eat. They climbed Ben Nevis, the highest peak in the British Isles, but by the time they reached Inverness, Keats fell ill with a persistent cold and sore throat which forced him to return to England by sea.

Upon his arrival he found that Tom was extremely ill. Immediately he moved into the room occupied by his brother and took complete care of him, never leaving the bedside. Rain continued all through the early winter, and John kept the windows tightly closed, sharing with his contemporaries the belief that this was the best protection against disease. When a few years later he heard that his beloved Fanny Brawne was suffering from a bad cold, he anxiously wrote her to "be careful of open doors and windows." Although most English physicians did not then believe in the contagiousness of phthisis, Keats was probably somewhat aware of the danger entailed by constant and close association with his brother. His friend, John Severn, expressed to him the popular belief that anyone who spent long hours in the room of a dying consumptive was liable to be attacked by the same disease, and he urged him to take a room apart from his brother. Keats refused, but letters of this time reveal that he was not without apprehension. "I live now in a continual fever," he wrote, "it must be poisonous to life, although I feel well."

Keats often experienced an almost physical projection of his mind into other minds or objects, both the penalty and the reward of his sensitive nature. On certain occasions, the identity of other persons so pressed upon him as to make him share their emotions, problems and sufferings. "Even if a Sparrow come before my Window I take part in its existence and pick about the Gravel." Or again, "When I am in a room with people, if I ever am free from speculating on creations of my own brain, then not myself goes home to myself, but the identity of everyone in the room begins so to press upon me, that I am in a very little time annihilated." As his brother became weaker, John felt that his own life was ebbing away. Thus, while his body was being exposed to the microbial agents of infection, he seemed to surrender his mind to disease through his identification with his brother. Tom died in December, 1818, at the age of nineteen.

For John, 1819 was a bad year. The memory of Tom haunted him. His poetry was attacked by the reviewers. His financial difficulties were increasing. And he was deeply in love with the vivacious, high-spirited Fanny Brawne, yet there had been misunderstandings between them. At the end of June he parted from her to go to the Isle of Wight, but this did not quiet the pangs of his jealousy. Back in London, he continued to seek refuge and inspiration in nature, seemingly unaware of creeping illness. On a February day of 1820, he returned from a short trip, coatless on the top of a coach in cold, snowy weather. Chilled to the bone, he was seized by high fever, and became so flushed and nervous as to appear drunk. Getting into bed, he coughed and suddenly tasted blood in his mouth. "Bring me the candle," he called to Brown, with whom he was staying, "and let me see this blood." He looked at the bright red spot on his pillow and then, his excitement and intoxication gone, he said calmly, "I know the color of that blood. It's 'arterial' blood. . . . That blood is my death warrant, I must die." Brown ran for the surgeon, who, according to the honored medical practice of the day, bled John from the arm, the first of the many bleedings that were to hasten his course to the grave.

It was not in a romantic attempt to dramatize his fate that Keats had forecast his early death, but from precise and painful experience. He remembered his own mother dying of some ill-defined consumption, and more acute in his memory — indeed, in his very flesh — was his brother Tom spitting the death blood of the pulmonary phthisic.[3] In the course of his medical experience, he had seen countless young men and women become sick and go into a "decline." Often, this became a wasting consumption, the body burning away in a relentless fever; and in many patients the disease underwent its inexorable evolution to pulmonary phthisis, with a destruction of the lung that usually meant death.

And now there was on the pillow of John Keats, twenty-four years old, that telltale, brilliant red blood. It is probable that he had been agitated and in poor health long before this acute attack. "For six months before I was taken ill I had not passed a tranquil day," he wrote. Six months previous was the time of his first parting from Fanny Brawne.

During the following spring Keats suffered repeated pulmonary hemorrhages. Doctors continued to bleed him frequently from the arm — and believed that they were combatting the progress of the disease by keeping him on a starvation diet. In order to brighten his spirits, Armitage Brown had moved him onto a sofa bed in the living room; there Keats received visits, night and day, from his neighbors, and in particular spent many hours with Fanny Brawne.

Despite the progress of his disease, Keats now and then pretended to hope. He began to consider his doctor's advice that he escape from the inclement weather of England and move toward brighter skies. In August, 1820, he wrote to Leigh Hunt: "'Tis not yet consumption, I believe, but it would be were I to remain in this climate all winter; so I am thinking of either voyaging or traveling to Italy." Accompanied by his devoted friend, the young painter Severn, he started for Italy in September, 1820, aboard the *Maria Crowther*. She was a small cargo boat, equipped with one single cabin for the five passengers, and the sea voyage from London to Naples lasted six weeks. One of the occupants of the stuffy cabin was a pretty, gentle girl "very lady-like, but a sad martyr," also a consumptive, going in search of the Italian warmth and sunlight. Dangerously ill, she craved air and wanted the portholes wide open, but the sharp blast of air would cause Keats to cough violently and sometimes to bring up blood. When the porthole was again closed, it was the turn of the poor girl to suffer, and she fell victim to fainting spells. The food was generally bad, and often spoiled. For the sake of the two consumptives, the captain tried, without success, to get a goat on board, since goat milk was then in great repute for the treatment of consumption. The travelers were exhausted when they reached Naples. Keats found no strength to convey in words the beauty of the Bay, realizing for the first time the paralysis of his poetical powers. And, after the miserable sea voyage, there was still the strenuous trip by chaise before arriving in Rome.

On the advice of the most distinguished physician of the English colony, Dr. James Clark, and in the company of other English consumptives, Keats began to take exercise on horseback and to spend much time on the Pincian Hill. Dr. Clark still felt uncertain as to the diagnosis of his ailment, being inclined to regard it as a case of "gastric fever," involving the stomach rather than the lungs. During December, several hemorrhages and a continuous high fever sapped Keats's strength to such an extent that he was compelled to inactivity. As in England, his physician added to the misery of the disease by taking blood from the arm and keeping him on the cruelly low diet of a single anchovy and a morsel of bread. Keats complained bitterly of these "pseudo victuals," feeling sure that "a mouse would starve upon it" and that he would die of hunger. Full of pity, Severn now and then brought him extra food, only to be warned by the doctor that he would kill his friend by exceeding the prescribed diet.

Frightened by consumption, the Italian landlady and her maid would do nothing to help. Severn had to make the beds, light the fire, and fetch the food by himself, compelled now and then, we are told, to have it pulled up through the window. Wanting to move the invalid into a larger and sunnier room, he found that the Italian law decreed the burning of all the furniture and objects present in lodgings that had been occupied by a consumptive. To escape the ordeal, Severn moved his friend without the knowledge of the landlady, trying to ease by a more cheerful environment the suffering caused Keats by disease and by the haunting memory of Fanny Brawne.

It was all to no avail. Keats knew that death was coming and, anxious for his devoted friend, begged him not to jeopardize his own health. "You must not look at me in my dying gasp, nor breathe my passing breath — not even breathe on me." On February 23, 1821, Keats died peacefully, as in his sleep. The following day autopsy showed the lungs to be almost entirely destroyed, his physician wondering how he had managed to survive during the last few months.

It was only one year since Keats had recognized the bright red blood on his pillow. To him, as to the medical knowledge of his time, this was the first sign of the disease. But almost certainly the hemorrhage had been only the eruption revealing a process which had long been smoldering in the dark, and which had begun at the bedside of Tom or perhaps even earlier.

On hearing of the passing of Keats, Shelley wrote in homage to his fellow poet verses glorifying the charm of young death:

> From the contagion of the world's slow stain
> He is secure, and now can never mourn
> A heart grown cold, a head grown gray in vain;
> Nor, when the spirit's self has ceased to burn,
> With sparkless ashes load an unlamented urn.

CHAPTER III

Flight from the North Winds

LIKE KEATS, Shelley was tuberculous and was soon to die under Italian skies. But it was accidental death, not disease, that spared him "a heart grown cold, a head grown gray in vain." The year 1817 had been difficult for him, tormented as he was by financial difficulties and by the consequences of his tragic relations with Harriet Westbrook. He felt ill, suffering from the stricture of pleurisy that later made him cry:

> I could lie down like a tired child,
> And weep away the life of care
> Which I have borne and yet must bear
> Till death like sleep might steal on me.

To Godwin he wrote:

> My health has been materially worse; my feelings at intervals are of a deadly and torpid kind, or awakened to a state of such unnatural and keen excitement, that, only to instance the organ of sight, I find the very blades of grass, the boughs of distant trees, present themselves to me with microscopical distinctness. . . . But I have experienced a decisive pulmonary attack; and although at present it has passed away without any very considerable vestige of its existence, yet this symptom sufficiently shows the true nature of my disease to be consumption. It is to my advantage that this malady is in its nature slow, and, if one is sufficiently alive to its advances, is susceptible of cure from a warm climate.

Accompanied by his wife and their children, he started for Italy in 1818, partly to escape the cold but also running away from a troubled life. Restless, they roved through Italy; their baby Clara died in Venice and their son William in Rome, both probably from enteric fevers. In Florence, Shelley's stabbing pain returned, and on his doctor's advice he moved on to the milder climate of Pisa. There, his health improved, but accidental drowning ended his life as he was sailing in the *Ariel.* A few days later, his decomposed body was found on the shore barely recognizable; two small volumes, one of Sophocles and one of Keats, were still in his jacket.

Keats and Shelley symbolize the romantic and consumptive youths of the nineteenth century, fleeing from melancholy skies and cold damp gloom. They were part of a great pilgrimage, begun long before, leading the sick from the Northern fog toward the Southern sun — the shrine of health, joy and illusion. As late as 1890, an article in the English *Review of Reviews* still referred to the Mediterranean coast as "the last ditch of the consumptive." Two full-page views of Monte Carlo and Monaco were accompanied by the comment, "It is a lovely country. But the cough of the consumptive is never still, even there."

In "Ordered South" Robert Louis Stevenson writes of the feeling of exhilaration experienced by the invalid at the mere thought of that "indefinable line that separates South from North." But this feeling rarely persisted after arrival in the promised land. Stevenson had observed that the invalid began to understand the change which had befallen him on discovering that his heart no longer could react spontaneously to the glory of nature. The consumptive was "like an enthusiast leading about with him a stolid, indifferent tourist." He could still realize beauty through his intelligence and memory, but no longer through his inward heart. It was in that somber mood that the glamorous and romantic heroes of the nineteenth century crowded under the sparkling sun and before the blue waters of the Riviera, feeling life withdraw and wither up from round about them.

Nice was the most fashionable rendezvous for those who tried to dodge death every winter by escaping from northern frosts.[1] At the Opera House, performances of the "cooing, phthisical" music of the Romantic Era nightly attracted throngs of corpse-like consumptives. The young women were smartly dressed and lavishly jeweled, but so pale beneath their curls that their faces appeared to be powdered with "scrapings of bones." Indeed, it seemed to one witness as if cemeteries were not closed at night and allowed the dead to escape.

It was in Nice that Nicolò Paganini, shaken by fits of coughing, reduced to a shadow, and with haunting, sunken features, came to spend his last winter in 1839.[2] Although syphilitic and consumptive since early manhood, the master of the violin had given throughout his life strenuous recitals all over Europe, adding the excitement of disorderly amorous adventures to the fatigue caused by extensive traveling and virtuoso playing. So thin was he that when he bowed to acknowledge applause the audience feared to see his frame fall apart as a heap of bones. Tuberculosis of the larynx had stilled his voice, and his young son, who always accompanied him on his travels, could hear his whispered words only by climbing onto a chair and placing his ear close to his father's mouth. Prolonged periods of agonizing illness often postponed his concerts and many of his astounding technical feats were performed while he was suffering great pain. His cadaverous, satanical appearance contributed still more drama to his playing. Heine spoke of the violinist's face as "pallid and corpse-like. . . . Did that look of entreaty belong to one who was deathly sick, or did the mockery of a crafty money-grabber lurk behind it? Was that a man on the point of death, who wished with his convulsions to delight his audience in the *arena of art, like a dying gladiator?* Or was it a dead man risen from his grave, a vampire with a violin, who would surely suck the money from our pockets, if not the blood from our hearts?"[3]

Paganini blamed the climate of England, Germany and France

for the continuous decline of his health. He fled from death first to Marseilles, then to Genoa and finally to Nice; but death pursued him. The voice of his violin had not been stilled and on the last night of his existence, the mute violinist played a brilliant improvisation from his deathbed. He did not receive the last rites of the Catholic Church and his body was refused burial in sacred ground despite his son's protestations to the Bishop that "as in all cases of phthisis, the sufferer never believed his end was approaching, but had died suddenly."

A few years later it was Rachel, the "divine" actress, who came to beg of the Mediterranean sun a last ray of hope.[4] Elisa Rachel Félix was born in 1821, the daughter of an itinerant Jewish peddler. She was almost uneducated, avaricious, and uniformly unfaithful to her lovers. But she had brought to the French theater a new concept of the classical drama. Instead of the usual elevation of voice and loud outburst of grief, she uttered her words hoarsely and with a concentrated feeling that gave to her roles an intensity new to the audience. This style was in part calculation. But the frailty and fatigue caused by tuberculosis had also compelled her to adopt a technique of acting compatible with her physical limitations.

> She stood [wrote Charlotte Brontë], not dressed but draped in pale antique folds, long and regular like sculpture. A background, and entourage, and flooring of deepest crimson threw her out, white like alabaster — like silver — rather be it said, like death. Wicked, perhaps, she is, but also she is strong, and her strength has conquered beauty, has overcome grace, and bound both at her side. . . . She disclosed power like a deep, swollen winter river, thundering in cataract, and bearing the soul like a leaf, on the steep and stately sweep of its descent.

In 1855 Rachel had been playing *Les Horaces* with her French troupe in New York when she fainted as the curtain fell. She persisted in her tour but caught a severe cold and collapsed again a few days later in Philadelphia. Ordered to the milder climate of Charleston, she appeared there on the stage in December, 1855, in what proved to be her last public performance. She knew that the end was coming — "I have done with illusions. I see myself already in the tomb." She proceeded to Havana, then to Egypt, holding court on her barge as she traveled up the Nile despite the progress of her malady. Back in Paris she realized that she was now a mere skeleton, a shadow of her past. "You who knew Rachel in the brilliance of her splendor and the riot of her glory, who have so often heard the theater ring with her triumphs — you would not believe that the gaunt spectre which now drags itself wearily over the world is — Rachel." With the approach of winter, she retired to Le Cannet, near Nice, where she lingered for a few weeks, white as snow, with burning eyes made brighter with fever. In January, 1858, she sank into a stupor following an attack of extreme suffocation. She died shortly after, at the age of thirty-eight, murmuring a line from *Les Horaces,* one of her greatest triumphs, and in her last breath calling the name of her favorite sister, Rebecca, who had died of tuberculosis four years before.

At the same period as Rachel, the Tsarevitch Nicholas, presumptive heir to the throne of Russia, was also receiving treatment for consumption in Nice. His mother visited him there on several occasions, and in 1865 the Tsar Alexander II came to receive his last words and to order the return of his body to Russia on board the frigate *Alexander Nevsky.*

To Nice also came, a few years later, the brilliant, hypersensitive and vain Marie Bashkirtsev.[5] Born in Russia in 1860, she had settled with her mother in Paris to study art. She began during early girlhood a detailed diary of her emotional life which achieved great and lasting fame when published, first in French, then in English, under the title, *The Journal of a Young Artist.* The stern Gladstone regarded it as "a book without a parallel."

"If I do not die young," wrote Marie Bashkirtsev in a revealing preface, "I hope to live as a great artist; but if I die young, I intend to have my Journal, which cannot fail to be interesting, published." She loved clothes, society, love, and yearned even more for glamour. Although sickly and fragile, she had unbounded energy, believing herself "made for triumphs and emotions." She decided to become a singer, but turned to painting when her voice, at first promising, was ruined by tuberculous laryngitis.

There was much tuberculosis in Marie's family and household. Her governess "was a sorrowful-looking creature, with her fifty years, and her consumption." Her father was "pale, delicate in health and the son of . . . a sickly mother, who died young." To the physician who diagnosed her disease, she affirmed that her grandfather, two of his sisters, a great-great-grandfather, and two grand-aunts had had consumption. Coughing, ailing much of the time, with pains in her side, she was seen by the most eminent physicians of the day. Suspecting that the fashionable doctors were concealing from her the true nature of the disease, she dressed in her maid's clothes and went to a clinic in one of the poorest sections of Paris, where she learned that both lungs were seriously affected. Marie's physicians, trying only mildly to restrain her burning eagerness, now ordered that blisters be applied to the chest and that she go South. While in Nice, she enjoyed the beauty of the city and was conscious of adding to its poetical charm as she walked about "silent and white as a shadow." But the attraction and glamour of Paris soon called her back to the capital, where she died at the age of twenty-four in October, 1884, mentioning, in her last breath, her painting at the Salon.[6]

The Brownings and the Trollopes, sojourning in Florence for the sake of the consumptive members of their families, formed the nucleus of a large Anglo-Italian circle which also welcomed many Americans. Among them was David Home, a clergyman from Connecticut, who had been compelled by tuberculosis to leave the United States and give up the ministry. In Italy he devoted himself to spiritualism and became the most famous medium. His séances were the focus of attention of the circle and were followed with intense passion, in particular by Elizabeth Browning.

An Englishwoman, Mrs. Carleton, published *Brief Advice to Travellers in Italy, Addressed to Persons who Travel for the Purpose of Health, Economy or Education.* Mrs. Carleton had very definite ideas about places of residence in the South. She warned that, despite its soft balmy air, the climate of Palermo was deceptive "and unfavorable to diseased lungs, being of an exciting nature, but in a less degree than the treacherous breeze of Naples, which may be called irritating." Nice, she felt, was agreeable but not safe as it caused the invalid's complaints to shift about mysteriously.

> Even individuals from that most guessing nation, America, have found that they were mistaken in their calculations. . . . The effect of a certain situation on the constitution depends in some degree upon the nature of the place from whence one *comes.* Thus a person whose system has been too much lowered at Rome will recover at Naples — one coming from Switzerland or Germany will find the nervous action let down to the right point at Rome, while an East Indian will complain that it is too relaxing. The *length of time* that a person remains is also a matter of consideration — one who arrives with a good provision of nervous excitement may feel well for several years at Rome, and when this is expended, some of the functions may become torpid, the liver may become clogged, and a journey to Naples may become necessary. The climate in all these cases remains intrinsically the same; let me not therefore be accused of incorrectness, if the effect of my climate does not always answer expectations.

Mrs. Carleton stated that the Sicilians' belief in the contagiousness of phthisis led them to take extravagant and bizarre precautions. She had little faith in continental physicians, warning that "it is rare to find out of England a physician whose superior sagacity enables him to handle an English patient without killing him." So unchangeable are national prejudices in medical matters!

In the New World, also, the "lungers" looked to milder climates for salvation. A few, wealthy and enterprising enough, crossed the Atlantic to Europe. At least one of them, Washington Irving, who had gone abroad to cure an "inflammation of the lungs," returned with health and with fame. But for most Americans, the Southern and Western states were less forbidding than Europe. Florida and the Caribbean Islands, and later Colorado, New Mexico and Arizona, provided for the North American consumptives the illusion of refuge with which the Mediterranean lured their European brothers in disease.[7]

So large, in fact, was the trek of consumptives to the South that many odd traces of it are found in the literature of the time. In *East Angels* Constance Fenimore Woolson has much to say concerning the Northerners ordered to St. Augustine for consumption. The poet, Sidney Lanier, himself a victim of the disease, had moved all over the South in search of a favorable climate.[8] While in Florida, he wrote a guidebook with special advice for the consumptive: "Set out to get well, with the thorough assurance that consumption is curable." The fundamental principle in treatment is "the making of the body as strong as possible by food, drink, air and physical development. Never get in the slightest degree wet, cold or tired." Although Lanier was in favor of some alcoholic stimulants, he advised that they be taken in amounts sufficiently small as neither to quicken the pulse nor to produce any sensation in the legs. "As between dying a drunkard and dying a consumptive, no one in his senses could hesitate a moment in favor of the latter alternative." More unexpected is the advice that he gave consumptives to help them earn a living in Florida. Along with some interest in farming activities, he recommended to those fond of woods-life that they shoot herons for their plumes or kill alligators and sell their teeth – which, at the price of four to ten dollars a pound, found a good market in the making of whistles or watch charms. In spite of all his optimism and sensible opinions, Lanier himself died of tuberculosis at the age of thirty-nine in Lynn, North Carolina.

In retrospect, it is difficult to understand the medical justification for the long and difficult travel urged on consumptives from Northern countries to the Mediterranean shores or to Florida. There was, certainly, a sense of well-being and euphoria that quickened the pulse of those arriving under the Southern skies after having left the depressive clouds of late fall and winter in the North. For many Northerners, the South also meant escape from worries and responsibilities. There were, furthermore, many records of spectacular recovery. Such was the case of Cecil Rhodes.[9] While studying for the Church in Oxford, his health had broken and at the age of sixteen he was sent to join his elder brother, then ranching under the luminous skies of Natal. That year diamonds were discovered in the Kimberley fields, and Cecil Rhodes found, in Natal, not only renewed vigor but also an immense fortune. Back in Oxford, after having walked through South Africa and determined that Britain should rule it, he became sick again in 1873 and was told that he had less than six months to live if he stayed in England. He returned to South Africa and, his health finally restored, settled again in Oxford in 1878.

Rhodes shared with many physicians the conviction that the hot, dry air of South Africa had saved him from consumption. But there were many others who believed that, in reality, the long sea voyage was responsible for the beneficial effects attributed to sojourning in southern climates. It was the custom in Imperial Rome to send those affected with diseases of the lung on a sea voyage to Sicily or Egypt. Cicero, gravely ill, coughing and expectorating blood, emaciated, his neck thin and flabby, and with hereditary predisposition to phthisis, had undertaken long voyages to Greece and Asia in 80 B.C. and had returned to Rome entirely cured two years later. And similarly, many English consumptives of the nineteenth century voyaged in Southern waters, encouraged by the memory of ancient medical traditions.

A notice of 1884 reports that the *Sobraon,* a sailing vessel of more than 2000 tons, had left the English coast with her load of consumptives bound for Australia through the Cape of Good Hope.[10] The eastbound voyage was to last three months and, after six weeks in Melbourne, the *Sobraon* was to sail west and bring her patients back to England. Although steamships could make the trip faster, sailing vessels were recommended because their slow tempo gave more time for adaptation to changes of temperature, and because they assured greater freedom from noise, smoke and fumes. Since sailing vessels presented the objection of exposing their passengers to some long stretches of hot, humid weather at the time of crossing the tropics, enterprising promoters planned to use auxiliary steam power to get quickly through the unfavorable regions. But this project did not materialize. For as the century came to an end, physicians and patients began to lose some of their faith in the power of the sun to cure consumption. It was painfully obvious to everyone that the White Plague recognized no geographical or climatic borders — killing young men and women just as effectively in Rome or Athens as in Paris or London, among the Polynesian Islanders as among the Transcendentalists of New England.

CHAPTER IV

Contagion and Heredity

UNIVERSAL as was the dread of consumption, it affected human behavior differently in various parts of the world. The diverse theories concerning the nature and spreading of the distemper determined the ways in which society tried to protect itself.

In certain countries the disease was regarded as catching, a contagion communicated through the air to the well person by some material emanating from the breath of the consumptive patient or from his belongings. In other places, by contrast, consumption was believed to be the product of a constitutional defect, often inherited from one's parents along with color of the hair or facial features.

The theory of contagion had been clearly expressed by a Florentine physician, Hyeronymus Fracastorius, in 1546. So great was the prestige of Italian learning that the theory was at first generally accepted throughout Europe, and indeed many striking facts were presented to support it. For example, there was reported in 1648 the story of three young Brandenburg counts who had contracted phthisis from their teacher, and in 1697 that of a physician said to have become consumptive because he was in the habit of tasting the sputum of his patients for diagnosis. As human milk was often prescribed for the treatment of consumption, a practice still in favor late in the nineteenth century even in the United States, there were stories of nurses having caught the disease from their patients. More incredible tales found credence. The celebrated physiologist Van Swieten stated that the kiss of a wife dying of phthisis took the hair off a spot on her husband's head. Panarolli, an Italian physician, was reported as having seen a man fall dead after stepping on the sputum of a consumptive, and another contract the disease after inhaling the fumes given off by sputum expectorated on burning coal.

So firm was the belief in contagion among Italian physicians of the eighteenth century that Giovanni Morgagni and other anatomists avoided performing autopsies on patients dead of phthisis in order to protect themselves and their students from contracting the disease. The most important consequence of the dread of contagion was to stimulate in Italy and Spain the enactment of regulations designed to prevent its spread. It was thus that in 1699 the Republic of Lucca promulgated the first decree of prophylaxis in the European annals of antituberculous legislation. The edict gave directives to protect the citizens from being "harmed or imperiled by objects remaining after death of a person suffering from phthisis," and it ordered physicians to "give notice of persons of either sex . . . treated for the suspected malady." The governing bodies of other Italian cities, and later Ferdinand VI of Spain, followed suit, the last edict being made in Naples.

The forceful statement by which a group of physicians of Naples recommended the new regulations to the Department of Health is not without interest. "Pulmonary consumption is of such a malignant nature in our country that even after the death of the sick person the seed of his malady remains hidden and unseen in many houses, with serious danger to those who move into them thoughtlessly; and indeed some of this seed is so penetrating that it can be communicated even without immediate contact with the infected person or thing."

The law ruled:

I. That the physician shall report a consumptive patient when ulceration of the lungs has been established. Failure to do so entails a penalty of three hundred ducats for the first offense and banishment for ten years for repetition of it.

II. That the authorities make an inventory of the clothing in the patient's room, to be identified after his death. In case of any opposition being made the person giving trouble shall have three years in the galleys or in prison, if he belongs to the lower class, and three years in the castle and a penalty of three hundred ducats if of the nobility.

III. That household goods not susceptible of contamination shall immediately be cleansed and those susceptible shall at once be burned and destroyed.

IV. That the authorities themselves shall replaster the house from cellar to garret, carry away and burn the wooden doors and windows and put in new ones.

V. That the poor sick shall at once be removed to a hospital.

VI. That newly built houses shall not be inhabited within one year after their completion and six months after the plastering has been done and everything about the building operation has been finished.

VII. That superintendents of hospitals must keep clothing and linens for the use of consumptives in separate places.

These regulations were enforced at first with relentless vigor, particularly in Spain. Indeed, it has been suggested that the thorough enforcement of the Spanish law against the emigration of consumptive individuals accounts for the fact that the Indians remained free of tuberculosis longer in the parts of America colonized by the Spaniards than in the parts colonized by the English and the French.

Soon, however, opposition developed everywhere, in part because certain physicians were not entirely convinced of the contagiousness of phthisis, in part because the strict application of the edicts was too costly, also because so many personal interests were involved. In Florence the edict was revoked in 1754, and in Naples a new, emasculated one was issued, merely trusting to "the diligence and care of the attending physician that he educate his phthisical patients to the wisdom of precautionary measures."

However, the revocation of the laws had not decreased the widespread belief in the catching nature of phthisis among the plain folk of Southern Europe, and there are many incidents which illustrate this dread of contagion.

In 1818, during one of his concert tours, Paganini suffered a severe relapse of his tuberculous disease, while in Naples. Convinced that any current of air was injurious to his health, he took a well-sheltered apartment below San Elmo. But his health daily became worse, and soon the landlord guessed the nature of the illness. Alarmed at having in his house someone suffering from the dreaded malady, he turned his tenant out into the street with all his possessions. Fortunately for Paganini, one of his friends happened to be passing by at the time and took him to more hospitable lodgings, not without first beating the frightened landlord with his stick.

A few years later, it was the French writer, René de Chateaubriand, who discovered at his expense that the fear of contagion was still alive in Italy. He had much difficulty finding a house to rent in Rome for his friend Madame de Beaumont, who was suffering from advanced phthisis. When compelled to put his equipage on sale in order to secure some funds, he found to his great surprise that he could find no buyers. The story is reported in one of his letters to a friend from whom he was asking a loan of money: "I had hoped to get some two thousand écus for my carriages. But according to a law from the time of the Goths, phthisis is officially considered to be contagious in Rome. And as Madame de Beaumont has been seen riding with me two or three times nobody wants to buy them." In fact, he was ordered to burn his carriages.

A more tragic fate befell Frédéric Chopin in Majorca, where he had gone in search of a mild climate.

> I have been sick as a dog the last two weeks; I caught cold in spite of 18 degrees C. of heat, roses, oranges, palms, figs and three most famous doctors of the island. One sniffed at what I spat up, the second tapped where I spat it from, the third poked about and listened how I spat it. One said I had died, the second that I am dying, the third that I shall die. . . . I can scarcely keep them from bleeding me. . . . All this has affected the Preludes and God knows when you will get them.

Soon the natives became aware of the fact that Chopin was consumptive and they refused to have anything to do with him or his party. George Sand, who accompanied him on this trip, has left a lively account of their ordeal.

> At very great cost, we had succeeded in establishing ourselves in Majorca, a magnificent country but most inhospitable.
>
> After a month there, poor Chopin's disease got worse, and we called in one, two, then three physicians – every one of them more asinine than the others and who spread through the Island the news that their patient was suffering from the lungs. The tale stirred up great terror. Phthisis is scarce in these climates and is regarded as contagious. . . . The owner of our small house threw us out immediately and started a suit to compel us to replaster his house on the pretext that we had contaminated it.
>
> We went to take residence in the disaffected monastery of Valdemosa . . . but could not secure any servants, as no one wants to work for a phthisic. . . . We begged of our acquaintances that they give us some help – only one, the first, the last service! – a carriage to take us to Palma, from where we wanted to take a ship back home. But even this was refused us, although our friends all had carriages and wealth.
>
> We had to go three leagues through deserted side roads in "birlocho," that is, in wheelbarrows.
>
> When we arrived in Palma, Chopin had a terrifying hemorrhage; the following day, we boarded the only steamship that comes to the island and which is used to transfer pigs

> to Barcelona. There was no other way to move out of this wretched country.
>
> At the time of leaving the inn in Barcelona, the innkeeper wanted us to pay for Chopin's bed under the pretext that it was infected and that the police had given him orders to burn it.

Doubt as to the contagiousness of phthisis had been expressed by the Faculty of Paris around 1650. From there it soon spread over all Northern Europe. Northern physicians seem to have been led to believe that the disease was due to a constitutional hereditary defect rather than to contagion by the fact that it was particularly common and severe in certain families.

They had noticed, for example, that brothers and sisters often became consumptive at almost the same age. In 1688 Richard Morton wrote in his *Phthisiologia* the story of a Mr. Hunt, a citizen of London who had "lived almost from his youth to the seventieth year in a consumptive State, doing his business well enough by taking care." He had three sons, who all lived until they were about thirty, at "which time they were all, one after another, seized by the same inheritance with a consumption occasioned by Passions of the Mind and the drinking of Spirituous Liquors . . . the Distemper carried them all off before the emaciated old man died." More than a century later, Antoine Portal reported that in a family of Gaillac in the southeast of France all five children had reached the age of twenty-eight to thirty in perfect health, only to die of phthisis by the age of thirty-two; the first three had died within two years, and the last two some ten years later within six months of one another.[1]

History offers many examples of celebrated tuberculous families, the French royal Bourbon family being one of them. Louis XIII died of galloping consumption, his autopsy revealing extensive intestinal lesions and pulmonary cavities. His wife, Anne d'Autriche, also suffered from phthisis. Their son Louis XIV had long suffered from fistula of the fundament, probably of tuberculous origin, and was operated for it by the surgeon Felix. It is told that after the operation the courtiers applied dressings to themselves so that they could imitate His Majesty's limp! As the operation was successful, and the royal anus cured, Felix received a farm and 300,000 livres, in addition to being created Seigneur de Stains.

The literary world of the nineteenth century provides many well-documented examples of familial phthisis, but none is more dramatic than the case of the Brontës.[2] The Reverend Patrick Brontë was born in 1777 (on Saint Patrick's Day) of a poor family in County Down, Ireland. After much struggle, he succeeded in going to Cambridge for his education and in being ordained to a curacy. He married Maria Branwell of Cornwall in 1812 and had six children, all born during the following seven years. Mrs. Brontë's health was failing when the family moved to Haworth in Yorkshire in 1820. She died the following year at the age of thirty-eight, of some vague ailment that was diagnosed an "internal cancer."

There is much that is obscure in the personality of the Reverend Patrick Brontë. His rise from a poor farm background in Ireland shows that he did not lack ability and enterprising spirit. But in Haworth, he kept himself and his family aloof from the village folk as if the humble social surroundings of his parish did not satisfy some unavowed ambitions. He professed and practiced extreme austerity of life, believing that his children should be brought up simply and hardily. There were no carpets in the parsonage except in the parlor, despite the cold dampness of the stone floors and stairs; little or no meat was served at table, and the Reverend forbade his wife and children to wear any colorful clothes or silk dresses that might lead to personal vanity. Yet there are vague rumors that he had changed the family name from Brunty to Brontë when he moved from Ireland, and he was wont to display before certain strangers a front of charm and brilliance not in keeping with his restraint in everyday behavior.

Throughout his life he wore an enormous white stock which completely swathed his throat, justifying this seeming vanity by the perpetual bronchitis of which he was victim, and by the necessity of shielding his throat from the cold. The cravat extended to the tip of his chin, reaching to the ear lobes. As he wore it even during the hottest weather, one may wonder whether it did not serve some purpose other than protection from the elements, perhaps to hide the swollen nodes of scrofula. He took most of his meals alone on the pretext that he was suffering from digestive trouble, and liked to go on long walks by himself. He displayed little interest in his children—except in his son Branwell, upon whom he doted—keeping so aloof from the emotional life of his daughters that he learned of their literary efforts only after their books had been published.

It is in this strange environment that the six Brontë children developed in close association. Hand in hand, they roamed throughout their beloved moors, returning to play or read together in the tiny room which was their allotted "study." While wild winds and driving rains lashed the tombstones in the graveyard surrounding the parsonage, their imaginations colonized fanciful islands and kingdoms. When the time came for the oldest girls to receive a more formal education, Maria, Elizabeth, Charlotte and Emily, then aged eleven to seven, were sent to a semicharitable institution for the daughters of clergymen. It was this school that emerged later from the memory of Charlotte as the Lowood School in *Jane Eyre.* According to Charlotte's description, the boarders were always cold and hungry, the food was usually spoiled or burnt, the milk tainted, the supper nothing more than a thin oatcake and a drink of water taken from a common mug by all the tablemates. At night the "pale thin girls" slept two in a bed, and during exercise time they went into the low, damp garden. They herded together for shelter and warmth in the veranda "and . . . as the dense mist penetrated to their shivering frames, I heard frequently the sound of a hollow cough."

During January, a few months after the arrival of the Brontë girls at the school, there broke out among the pupils a terrifying epidemic described under the name of "typhus" in *Jane Eyre.* However, the disease was certainly something else, according to the account given by Charlotte to her friend, Mrs. Gaskell. The patients appeared too "dull and heavy to understand remonstrances, or to be roused by texts and spiritual exhortation." The disease "caused them to sink away into dull stupor and half-unconscious listlessness." "All heavy-eyed, flushed, indifferent and weary with pains in every limb" they lay about, "resting on tables or the ground." Although some forty of the girls suffered from the distemper, only one of them died of it, and her death occurred somewhat later after a lingering process. None of the Brontë sisters developed the disease in its acute form. But Maria and Elizabeth, twelve and eleven years old respectively, soon went into a decline, and had to be sent home – where they died in the following May and June.

The three remaining sisters and their brother Branwell spent most of the following six years at Haworth, apparently happy and beginning to write poetry and interminable fantasies. In 1831 Charlotte was sent as a pupil to a girls' school at Roe Head, and four years later she returned there as a teacher. At that time, Emily joined her as a pupil, but soon became literally ill of homesickness. "Every morning," wrote Charlotte, "the vision of home and the moors rushed on her, and darkened and saddened the day. Her white face, attenuated form and failing strength threatened rapid decline. I felt in my heart she would die if she could not go home." Emily returned to Haworth, and the youngest sister, Anne, joined Charlotte at Roe Head. But Anne soon developed a cough, with difficulty in breathing and a pain in her side. Frightened Charlotte, remembering the symptoms of Maria and Elizabeth, returned home with Anne and settled again at the Haworth parsonage.

In the course of the following years the three sisters left home on a few occasions to go to school as pupils or as governesses, but always with disastrous results to their health and morale. Only at Haworth did their natures expand. They longed for each other's company and for the presence of their brother as much as for the moors. Feverishly they pursued their literary work and soon succeeded in having their first writings published. The poetry and novels of the three sisters remained almost unnoticed until the appearance of *Jane Eyre,* which established Charlotte in the literary world. It was only after Emily's death that her poetry and *Wuthering Heights* achieved recognition.

Yet, it was in Branwell, his poetry and painting, that the hopes of the family were centered. The brilliance of his conversation was the pride of the Haworth pub, and all those who met him were charmed by his manner. Soon, however, Branwell became more and more self-indulgent, his debts mounted, and his attempts in any occupation ended in failure. While a tutor in a private home, he fell recklessly in love with the mother of his charges and had to return to Haworth in disgrace. From then on he became increasingly addicted to alcohol and opium, taking to the drug in order to quiet the endless coughing during his sleepless nights. Though obviously consumptive, he never was confined to bed and continued to the end his dissipated life in the village.

Branwell's behavior, illness and death in September, 1848, filled the Haworth parsonage with gloom. A sharp autumn wind blew upon the family as they followed the coffin to the cemetery, and the cold which Emily caught at that time became steadily worse. Her emaciation, persistent cough, painful breathing and racing pulse were the all too familiar signs of consumption. But still she refused to see a physician or to remain in bed, and she went about her household tasks as usual with "catching rattling breath and a glazed eye." She died at the age of twenty-nine, three months after Branwell.

Less than two weeks later, the local doctor diagnosed that frail Anne was suffering from advanced consumption, and he ordered a treatment including cod-liver oil and carbonate of iron. Full of anxiety, Charlotte sent a detailed account of her sister's symptoms to Dr. Forbes, an eminent London physician who had recently introduced Laënnec's stethoscope in England. Forbes's reply left little hope of a cure, but he approved of the cod-liver oil, which he held to be an efficacious remedy. Anne believed that her health could still be benefited by removal to a better climate and, accompanied by Charlotte, she left for the seaside at Scarborough, only to die four days later in May, 1849. She was then twenty-seven years of age.

Charlotte returned alone to the ghost-filled Haworth parsonage. Although she never enjoyed good health and mentioned with increasing frequency the pain between her shoulders, the cough that never left her, the sore throat and fever that killed her appetite and increased her thirst, she continued to write her novels until she married in 1854. Fame had not overcome her timidity, and though she was invited and feted in literary circles, she felt unhappy away from Haworth and among strangers. Soon after her marriage and early in the course of pregnancy, she developed a severe cold following a walk in the rain. A few months later, in 1855, she died, at the age of thirty-nine.[3]

The Reverend Patrick Brontë survived his wife and six children and lived to the age of eighty-nine. The death certificate ascribed his end to "chronic bronchitis." It is more likely that his bronchial irritation was of tuberculous origin and that he had been the source of the infection which had destroyed his entire family. His strange personality, and the confinement of his children during their early years within the narrow walls of the parsonage, may also have been influential in transmuting into poetry and novels the tragedies of which he had been the primary cause.

The family made famous by Ralph Waldo Emerson provides a typical example of familial tuberculosis in America.[4] Thomas Emerson came from England and settled in Ipswich, Massachusetts, in 1638. There is nothing in the history of the Emersons or of their wives to suggest that phthisis was a cause of illness or death among them during the first one hundred and fifty years of their stay in the Bay State. The children were mostly long-lived, except for those who died in infancy, a frequent occurrence in those days when enteric fevers were prevalent. The first unquestionable case of pulmonary consumption occurs in the fifth generation. Reverend William Emerson died of the disease in 1811, at the age of forty-two. There is no evidence that he had been exposed to a case of tuberculosis in his household, and it has been presumed that he acquired the infection while at college, where he led a frugal and strenuous life, or in the course of his pastoral duties to which he devoted himself unsparingly. This was a time when consumption was the most frequent of the recognized causes of death in New England and particularly in Boston.

William's widow, Ruth Emerson, was left with five boys and an infant daughter, and no financial resources. But she accepted the challenge of self-support and the sacrifice of physical comfort for the sake of high moral and intellectual achievement. "If a precious book were needed for school or college studies the coal oil for the hall lamp could be given up. Better a dark hall than a starved mind."

The infant daughter had died of unknown cause shortly after her father, and one of the sons, not mentally strong, was to die of some cause other than tuberculosis at the age of fifty-two. The other four boys, William, Ralph Waldo, Edward Bliss and Charles Chauncy, went to Harvard and graduated with high academic honors between the years 1818 and 1828. But this was bought at the cost of great privation.

> It is told that one winter overcoat had to serve in turn in bitter weather, only one of the collegians being in attendance at Cambridge on such days to take lecture notes for the others not clad to meet a north-east snow storm, footing it over the Charles Street bridge. Stories of the Greek heroes were read aloud to the younger boys by their mother when on some days food was scarce and attention had to be temporarily diverted from inner hunger.

All four boys developed tuberculosis. The eldest, William, showed signs of pulmonary disease during early adulthood and passed through several episodes of illness during the rest of his life. For many years he suffered from winter "bronchitis," but lived to the age of sixty-seven, when he died of pneumonia. Ralph Waldo also had suffered from pulmonary tuberculosis while at Divinity School in Boston. He knew then that "a mouse was gnawing at his chest." In the autumn of 1826 new symptoms of disease made it advisable that he close the school where he was teaching and, with the help of some funds obtained from his uncle, he decided to go South to escape the "northeast winds." But even Charleston proved too cold for his lungs. He felt "not sick, not well, but luke-sick." "Oppressions and pangs chiefly by night" disturbed him, also "a certain stricture on the right side of the chest, which always makes itself felt when the air is cold or damp." He proceeded to Florida and finally returned to Boston, not completely cured. Throughout his life he complained of a bronchitis, certainly the manifestation of chronic phthisis. But he overcame the acute form of his disease and lived to the age of seventy-nine.

However, tuberculosis claimed many lives around him. During the summer of 1834 his brother Edward Bliss died of galloping consumption in Puerto Rico after an accidental wetting had intensified his chronic cough, and in 1835 his other brother,

Charles Chauncy, then 27, died in New York, also of galloping consumption. But it was in the illness of his first wife, Ellen, that Ralph Waldo suffered the blow that probably left the most indelible stamp on his future life.

Ellen Louisa Tucker of Concord, New Hampshire, was seventeen when he first met her in 1827. Her father, a prosperous merchant, died at the age of forty-seven. Five years later her brother George, then a medical student traveling abroad for health, died in Paris of "a horrid cold." Her sister Mary died young, and her other sister, Margaret, was certainly a victim of consumption. Emerson married Ellen in September, 1829. She had active pulmonary tuberculosis at the time of their marriage, and soon a "decline" compelled her to go South. Taking opiates to quiet her cough, she went horseback riding day after day, believing that exercise in the balmy open air was her last chance for life. But, as with so many others, the sun could not prevent the destruction of her lungs, and in January, 1831, she died.

Ralph Waldo married again in 1835, and four children were born of his second marriage. Tuberculosis continued to strike among his descendants as well as among those of his elder brother, William. In fact, a historical survey published in 1949 by a distinguished physician, grandson of the latter, reveals that tuberculosis has been the cause of several deaths and many cases of clinical illness up to and including the tenth generation of the Emerson family in this country. Yet it appeared that, at the time of writing, the oncoming generation, the eleventh, was still free of the disease.

Henry David Thoreau, also, was from a consumptive family.[5] His grandfather had died, consumptive, in 1801. In 1841 Henry's brother John showed signs of severe pulmonary disease but died the following year from lockjaw contracted in an accident. His sister Helen died in 1849, having been consumptive from girlhood.

His father died in 1859 after a sickness of several years during which, according to Thoreau's *Journal,* "he had coughed and expectorated a great deal."

Henry had many colds as a youth and during adulthood usually suffered from severe bronchitis in the late winter. His disease took a turn for the worse in the spring of 1856, but he forced himself for a while to continue his strenuous walks through the Concord country. By June, however, he had to confess that he was unwell, and he spent an inactive summer at Cape Cod. Although he was again able to resume fairly normal physical activities in the autumn, he never regained his former vigor.[6]

From then on, the paralyzing effect of advancing phthisis seems to be reflected in the mood of his *Journal.* Before his illness, the pages overflow with a passionate, almost inebriated, sense of the beauty of nature, stimulated by bodily contact with the fields, woods, rivers and lakes of Concord. After the waning of his physical vigor, the entries deal more and more with minute and dry records of detailed observations and with uninspired plans for a history of Indian life—as if a lack of vitality had stilled his creative genius. Late in 1860 he contracted a cold which marked the beginning of his last illness, and he abandoned his *Journal* after becoming confined to the house. In May he went to Minnesota, which was then a popular place for the treatment of consumptives. But he returned to Concord in October, his health unimproved. For a few months he lingered on, stretched on a sofa in the living room, where he spent his days receiving the visits of his friends. To the end he displayed a cheerful stoicism, refusing opiates even though he could not sleep. He died gently in May, 1862, at the age of 45.

This frequency of multiple cases of pulmonary consumption in one household, and the extinction of many consumptive families, made it appear certain in the Northern countries that the disease was the outcome of a bad hereditary constitution. It was generally considered that little could be done for those born with a predisposition to phthisis beyond providing for them a climate and a way of life that would retard the inexorable course of their disease. Only balmy air and sunny skies, it was thought, could arrest the destruction of lung tissue and the sapping of strength that otherwise drove the consumptive to certain death in the space of a few years.

CHAPTER V

Consumption and the Romantic Age

EPIDEMICS have often been more influential than statesmen and soldiers in shaping the course of political history, and diseases may also color the moods of civilizations. Because they are part of everyday life, however, their role is rarely emphasized by historians. Yet some aspects of the medical past which have remained almost unnoticed may have been of greater historical consequence than more celebrated events.

Whereas the influence of bubonic plague is obvious in Boccaccio's tales, and in the dissolution of morals at certain periods of the Renaissance, the part played by tuberculosis in more recent history is less distinct even though it was profound and lasting. The disease distorted the norms of life and behavior for several generations by killing young adults or ruining their physical and mental health.

Many of the pre-Romantics in the late eighteenth century appear to have been tuberculous.[1] According to their own memoirs, Jean Jacques Rousseau and Goethe both suffered from lung hemorrhages in their early adulthood, and it is known of Laurence Sterne, Friedrich Schiller, Novalis, Ludwig Holty, Carl Maria von Weber, and Charles Hubert Millevoye that they died of phthisis. Tuberculosis, being then so prevalent, may have contributed to the atmosphere of gloom that made possible the success of the "graveyard school" of poetry and the development of the romantic mood. Melancholy meditations over the death of a youth or a maiden, tombs, abandoned ruins, and weeping willows became popular themes over much of Europe around

1750, as if some new circumstance had made more obvious the ephemeral character of human life. Instead of singing of the healthy joys of love, poets cultivated the refined sadness evoked by the thought that the beloved might soon depart. For Thomas Lovell Beddoes, whose father had written a famous *Essay on Consumption,* the earth was a "grave-paved star."

Ever since antiquity and through classical times, autumn had been depicted in literature as the time of bountiful harvests, the mellow season when men rejoiced in health and abundance. But this began to change around 1760. The sadness of autumn entered poetry.[2] Falling leaves came to symbolize discouragement and the destruction of young lives. In fact, not a few of the despairing poets were refused the joys of the harvest through early death. Holty, dying of consumption at the age of twenty-nine in 1776, compared his life to a rose "withered and carried by the wind." In "The Fall of the Leaves," Millevoye regarded the mournful hue of autumn as a forewarning of his own doom. He died consumptive at the age of thirty-nine, in 1816. Lamartine was more fortunate and survived by half a century the poems in which he took leave of the world. However, he too had suffered from chest disease in his late teens. It was while recovering near the Lac d'Annecy that he met Julie Charles who was there curing "a disease of languor." Julie, whom he immortalized later as Laurence in *Jocelyn,* Julie in *Raphael* and Elvire in *Meditations,* died of tuberculosis shortly after her return to Paris in 1817. The romantic love that she inspired in the poet led him to associate in his melancholy verses the foliage of autumn with the passing of life and the mourning of nature.

To Shelley the colors in fall, the pungent odors of woods and fields, the exhilarating crisp air, evoked only disease and death:

> O Wild West Wind, thou breath of Autumn being,
> Thou, from whose unseen presence the leaves dead
> Are driven, like ghosts from an enchanter fleeing,
> Yellow, and black, and pale, and hectic red,
> Pestilence-stricken multitudes . . .

And his poem "To Autumn" Shelley entitled "a dirge":

> The warm air is failing, the bleak wind is wailing,
> The bare boughs are sighing, the pale flowers are dying,
>   And the Year
> On the earth her death-bed, in a shroud of leaves dead,
>   Is lying.

Several decades later autumn still meant to William Cullen Bryant that . . .

> The melancholy days have come, the saddest of the year,
> Of wailing winds, and naked woods, and meadows brown
>   and sear.

It is this heaviness of heart that led the consumptive Swiss philosopher, Henri Amiel, to infect nature figuratively with his own disease after strolling in his garden under a fine rain. On an October day of 1852, he wrote in his *Journal Intime:*

> . . . Sky draped in gray, pleated by subtle shading, mists trailing on the distant mountains; nature despairing, leaves falling on all sides like the lost illusions of youth under the tears of incurable grief. The earth strewn with brown, yellow and rusty leaves, the trees half bare. . . . The fir tree, alone in its vigor, green, stoical in the midst of this *universal phthisis.*

Also in 1852 Thoreau remarked, in his *Journal,* after seeing the first spotted maple leaves "with a greenish center and a crimson border": "Decay and disease are often beautiful, like . . . the hectic glow of consumption."

It would be naïve to see in the prevalence and severity of tuberculosis the single cause of the weeping romanticism that characterized the early nineteenth century.[3] But the death of young adults was so commonly the result of the disease that it could not but sharpen the heart-stabbing sense of the brevity of life. Even more perhaps it contributed to literature a number of symbols, images and moods, of great emotional force because they were then the expression of impacts received in everyday life.

The pervading presence of tuberculosis throughout society is reflected in all fields of literature. In *Dream of the Red Chamber*, the first realistic novel in the Chinese language to be acknowledged as literature, the symptoms of the tuberculous heroine Black Jade serve to highlight her emotional crises.[4] The best sellers of the Victorian Era abound in disease, and consumption provided a natural manner to dispose of a character and facilitate the plot. Even the most skillful novelists made use of such a convenient device, perfectly believable because the death of young people was a common occurrence. In *David Copperfield* Charles Dickens found it poetical and easy to let Little Blossom die gracefully without disfigurement, almost without any symptoms. Washington Irving depicted in *The Bride of the Village* a young girl passing into a romantic and hopeless decline at the thought that her lover was unfaithful to her. And in *Wuthering Heights* Emily Brontë allowed many characters to die of some form of consumption. When one of them, Frances Earnshaw, first appeared at Wuthering Heights for the funeral of her husband's father, everything seemed to delight her except the presence of the mourners. The mere sight of black stimulated in her a hysterical emotion.

> She felt so afraid of dying! I imagined her as little likely to die as myself. She was rather thin, but young, and fresh-complexioned, and her eyes sparkled as bright as diamonds. I did remark . . . that mounting the stairs made her breathe very quick, that the least sudden noise set her all in a quiver, and that she coughed troublesomely sometimes; but I knew nothing of what these symptoms portended, and had no impulse to sympathize with her.

In June, after she had given birth to a boy, the doctor recognized that Frances had been in a consumption for many months and prophesied that she would die before the winter. A few days later, as she was telling her husband of her intention to get up the next day, a fit of coughing took her — a very slight one. He raised her in his arms, she put her two hands about his neck, her face changed, and she was dead.

Colds which settled obstinately on the lungs, fits of coughing, all kinds of fever — slow at their commencement, but incurable and rapidly consuming toward the close — were mysterious ailments which appeared frequently in the Victorian novel. But disease was rarely presented as something loathsome, unless it affected the villain. Rather, it was used as a device to enlist the sympathies of the reader. Consumption served the purpose well since it was believed to affect chiefly sensitive natures, and conferred upon them a refined physical charm before making them succumb to a painless, poetical death.

> Ay, thou art for the grave; thy glances shine
> Too bright to shine long; . . .
> And they who love thee wait in anxious grief
> Till the slow plague shall bring the fatal hour.
> Glide softly to thy rest, then; Death should come
> Gently, to one of gentle mood like thee,
> As light winds wandering through groves of bloom
> Detach the delicate blossom from the tree.
> Close thy sweet eyes, calmly and without pain.[5]

Thus, a decline could be used at will to render the heroine more attractive, to purify her soul through suffering and resignation, to show the cruel workings of an inevitable fate or to deal in fiction with vague problems of heredity and predestination.

Like their English and American counterparts, many of the romantic heroines of French literature during the nineteenth century were consumptive and died young. The model for Marguerite Gauthier, in *La Dame aux Camélias,* was Alphonsine

Plessis, born in 1824 in Normandy. She had illicit love affairs soon after leaving the village of her birth, but had retained throughout her life a childlike religious faith despite the vagaries of her existence. While still young, she had changed her name from Alphonsine to Marie, selecting the name of the Virgin because she thought it suitable to the pure expression of her own beautiful eyes. It was under the name of Marie Duplessis that she married a young and wealthy Englishman who died shortly after of tuberculosis.

Once more in Paris, she became one of the fashionable courtesans of the day, and met the playwright Alexandre Dumas *fils*. Their liaison lasted but a few months. While in a state of advanced pulmonary consumption, and despite her physicians' advice, she continued, to the end, a whirlwind of social life, seeking at the balls every night an escape from solitude. She was the center of worshiping attention wherever she went, and when she died in 1847, at the age of twenty-three, the public sale of her belongings was a social event. According to Charles Dickens, who attended the sale in Paris, one could have believed that Marie was a Jeanne d'Arc or some other national heroine, so profound was the general sadness.

Dumas learned of the death of his former mistress upon returning from a journey in Spain, and it appears that he wrote *La Dame aux Camélias* under the influence of the immediate emotion. The play enjoyed an enormous success. Such was the appeal of the theme that it became the custom for lovers to take camellias to the grave of Marie Duplessis in Paris; however, it seems that the use of the flowers in the play was purely imaginative, and that they had never been associated with the heroine during her life — as Dumas himself has testified. The play was seen in Paris by the American actress, Jean (Lander) Davenport, who insisted that it be immediately translated into English so that she might take the leading role. Under the title *Camille, or the Fate of a Coquette,* it was an even greater triumph in New York than in Paris, and its plot, hardly modified, was taken up in other plays and novels. Verdi utilized the theme in *La Traviata,* and when the opera was produced in Venice, in 1853, it rocketed the author to the front place among Italian composers.[6]

The original of Mimi of the opera *La Bohème* also lived in Paris of the 1840's. She was a flower girl of humble origin, married to a poor shoemaker. Seeking adventure and romance, she had followed a young architect, who had introduced her to a group of unconventional and impecunious artists and writers. They met as an informal club which was called Bohemia and of which Henri Murger was one of the leaders. Murger's verve and sentimentality appealed to the fickle Mimi and, despite his poverty, she came to live with him in 1847. She was already very ill, and after a year had to be taken to the Hôpital de la Piété, where she died of tuberculosis in 1848. In the same year, Murger achieved literary success with his novel *Scènes de la Vie de Bohème.* In 1849, the book was made into the play *La Bohème,* which later served as the basis for Puccini's opera. Thus, like Marie Duplessis, the facile and irresponsible Mimi indirectly determined the international fame of a writer and of a musician.

Tuberculosis appears frequently in one allusion or another in *Scènes de la Vie de Bohème.* For example, when Schaunard, the musician of the group, presenting himself as a concert pianist to a potential patron, assures him, "I would be as famous as the sun if I had a black suit, wore long hair, and if one of my lungs were diseased." Francine was another of Murger's consumptive heroines who, like Mimi, was "pale like the angel of phthisis." When told of her disease and warned that she might die with the falling leaves, she replied, "Why should the falling leaves worry us; let us spend our days among pine trees where leaves are always green." When Francine was compelled by weakness to remain in bed after October, her lover placed a curtain over the window to hide the tree that was losing its leaves in the courtyard. In November "a sharp wind blew onto her bed a yellow leaf torn from the tree . . . she hid it under her pillows." It was the same theme that O. Henry exploited in his story, "The Last Leaf." In this case, the leaf was painted on the wall outside the bedroom window to protect the young woman from dying with the falling of the last leaf. There had been a change of fashion in disease during O. Henry's time. His heroine died, not in a slow decline, but of the more explosive pneumonia.

During the latter part of the nineteenth century, writers became more and more eager to present in their stories an accurate account of contemporary life and to explain their observations on the basis of available scientific knowledge. The brothers Edmond and Jules de Goncourt were pioneers in the new physiological school of writing. In order to obtain firsthand documentation, they moved far and wide through the various social strata of Paris and recorded their impressions every evening in their famous *Journal.*

It is clear from many entries that the Goncourts often came into contact with the problem of phthisis, and were much intrigued by it. When they decided to spend some time at the Hôpital de la Charité to obtain material for their novel, *Sœur Philomène,* the first death that they had occasion to report was that of a phthisic forty years old whom they saw—"the mouth wide open, as that of a man who had expired while trying to breathe, without finding any air." And a few days later they witnessed an older man "with a bony and emaciated face, sunken eyes . . . shaking like an old dead tree blown by a winter wind," begging for care "with a soft, extinguished, slow and humble voice." Unable to admit the poor fellow and turning him out in the snow, the intern explained apologetically to his visitors, "if we accepted all the phthisics . . . we would not have any room left for other patients." Attending mass in the chapel of the hospital, the Goncourts noticed that the men and women patients sat by preference "on the side that showed their profile to the best advantage, for there were among them many with extensive scrofulous glands." Elsewhere they speak of their family servant, unexpectedly found to be consumptive. "The disease has worked quickly. One lung gone — the other about as bad." On August 11 she walked from her carriage to the hospital entrance; on August 16 she was dead. To their great surprise, they discovered after her death evidence of secret "nocturnal orgies . . . her consumption lending a sort of fury to her sensuality, a kind of hysteria, a beginning of madness." [7]

The Goncourts had personal reasons to be interested in tuberculosis, for one of their aunts had been consumptive and had died in Rome after becoming a religious fanatic. Believing that her abnormal psychic behavior was the outgrowth of pulmonary disease, they decided to treat the problem in a scientific novel. Its main character, Madame Gervaisais, was patterned after their aunt, and they undertook to describe objectively and in detail the symptoms and the psycho-physical evolution of her disease.[8] At one of the bimonthly dinners which it was their custom to attend, they heard a renowned physician, Dr. Robin, expose at length his views on the physiology of tuberculosis. The doctor believed that the disease brought about progressive modifications in the brain, which resulted in the mental characteristics peculiar to pulmonary phthisis. "What a pity, what a loss," wrote the brothers in their *Journal,* "that so intelligent an observer and physiologist should not write the book, of which he gave us so interesting a bit this evening, on the moral effects of diseases of the chest . . . a book which would be a medico-literary clinic . . . and would display all the revolutions of the soul in the sufferings of the body."

Having little faith in Dr. Robin's literary enterprise and talent, the brothers decided to incorporate his views in their own novel. Although *Madame Gervaisais* makes dull reading today, Emile Zola acknowledged it as one of his main sources of inspiration in formulating the doctrine of realism in the novel. In a kind of artless joinery, the Goncourts presented scenes illustrating the attitude toward tuberculosis in the nineteenth century: the Roman landlady fearful of accepting Madame Gervaisais as a tenant on discovering that she might be consumptive; the portly priest reading his *Benedicite* and suspicously pulling back his chair as from contact with a leper when he hears his pale neighbor ordering special food; the fashionable physician repeatedly bleeding his patients from the arm; the homeopath with his powders and ointments.

Madame Gervaisais is shown by the Goncourts with a "strange and exciting seduction . . . almost seraphic," that increased with the progress of her disease. The consumption which slowly destroyed her life transformed her into a mystical character, made her body aspire to "become a spirit, move toward the supernatural of spirituality."

> . . . The progressive disembodiment carried her ever more toward the saintly folly and the hallucinated joys of religious passion. She was driven to it through another effect of her illness. In contrast to the diseases of the crude, baser organs of the body, which clog and soil the mind, the imagination, and the very humors of the sick as though with corrupt matter, phthisis, this illness of the lofty and noble parts of the human being, calls forth in the patient a state of elevation, tenderness and love, a new urge to see the good, the beautiful and the ideal in everything, a state of human sublimity which seems almost not to be of this earth.[9]

This artificial description shows that, despite their efforts to describe life with realistic accuracy, the Goncourts did not escape the influence of their times. Like their contemporaries, they regarded tuberculosis as a refined disease in which the mind triumphs over the body. Their words hardly differ from those used by Charles Dickens in *Nicholas Nickleby:*

> There is a dread disease which so prepares its victim, as it were, for death; which so refines it of its grosser aspect,

> and throws around familiar looks, unearthly indications of the coming change — a dread disease, in which the struggle between soul and body is so gradual, quiet, and solemn, and the result so sure, that day by day, and grain by grain, the mortal part wastes and withers away, so that the spirit grows light and sanguine with its lightening load, and, feeling immortality at hand, deems it but a new term of mortal life; a disease in which death and life are so strangely blended that death takes the glow and hue of life, and life the gaunt and grisly form of death; a disease which medicine never cured, wealth never warded off, or poverty could boast exemption from; which sometimes moves in giant strides, and sometimes at a tardy sluggish pace, but, slow or quick, is ever sure and certain.

The distorted picture of consumption drawn by poets and novelists was in keeping with the peculiar ideal of feminine beauty that was then prevailing. In France, the boisterous female type of the Revolutionary era had been displaced in popularity shortly after 1800 by the languishing beauty dressed in vaporous muslins.[10] Sheer white materials of cotton, linen and silk became the rage, regardless of the season. The wearing of thin clothing, even during the winter, was in fact claimed by some hygienists of the time to be responsible for the influenza which broke out in Paris in 1803, and which was consequently referred to as the "muslin disease."[11] The new fashion was also believed, and is still considered in some modern writings, to have been instrumental in bringing on the epidemic of pulmonary phthisis that reached its peak shortly thereafter. When languid pallor became a fashionable attribute of women, the use of rouge was abandoned in favor of the whitening powders. It was not until the twentieth century that "sun-tan" powder appeared when glowing health became an attribute of beauty.

Edgar Allan Poe romantically satisfied the nineteenth-century pale ideal of feminine beauty through association with consumptive young women: first his child wife, Virginia; later Fanny Osgood, dying of a cough that was killing her "by inches, and there are not many inches left."[12] Various scenes of Virginia's life make of her the personification of the romantic heroine. One evening in January, 1842, the Poes were giving a party at their Fordham cottage. Dressed in white, "delicately, morbidly angelic," Virginia was singing and playing the harp in the glow of the lamplight. Suddenly she stopped, clutched her throat, and a wave of crimson blood ran down her breast. Although accidents such as this caused much anguish to Poe, he did not recognize hemorrhages of the lungs as evidence of severe pulmonary disease. Instead, he looked on his wife's illness as the source of a strange additional charm, which rendered more ethereal her chalky pallor and her haunted, liquid eyes.

Poe was not alone in regarding delicate women, given to fainting and languidly lying upon invalid couches, as the ideal of the poet. This attitude was so general that it secured a moment of literary fame for the now forgotten Davidson sisters of Plattsburg. Their mother, Mrs. Davidson, was a poetess and consumptive. Her two daughters, Lucretia and Margaret, published poetry which was widely acclaimed in America and England. Lucretia wrote in a dark room—to the music of an Aeolian harp in the window—strange and wild poems about the Near East; Margaret borrowed Western themes for her romantic outpourings. Both Lucretia and Margaret died of tuberculosis before they were twenty. Edgar Allan Poe, Washington Irving and the Poet Laureate, Robert Southey, wrote of them as the symbols of poetic fire, regarding consumptive death as a fitting climax to their genius.

To William Cullen Bryant, as to many others, the death of a beautiful girl was the most poetic of all themes—especially if she died in the fall, of some obscure, slow and wasting malady:

> We wept that one so lovely should have a life so brief,
> Yet not unmeet it was that one, like that young friend of ours,
> So gentle and so beautiful, should perish with the flowers.

The impact of consumption on nineteenth-century esthetics appears in the elongated "women with cadaverous bodies and sensual mouths" of the Pre-Raphaelite paintings.[13] The type had been personified first by Elizabeth Siddal, who married Gabriel Rossetti shortly before her death. Pale, with abundant red hair and long thin limbs, she served as model for ten years to several artists of the group. She posed notably for the "Ophelia" of Millais, in a splendid old dress with silver embroidery, drowning — for an hour at a time — in a bath filled with tepid water, not even protesting when the heating arrangement failed to function. Sad and silent, she was given to writing sentimental poems crowded with gray tombstones and the thought of death.

Elizabeth probably developed tuberculosis while still a young girl, and she was sickly throughout her short life. But the nature of her disease remained indefinite. Curvature of the spine, pulmonary phthisis, and "mental power long pent up and lately overtaxed" were the diagnoses of three different physicians who examined her between the ages of twenty-five and twenty-eight. Ruskin, who was fond of her, helped her financially to go for rest to the South of France and to Algeria. But she progressively failed in health and her mood saddened further. She died in London in 1864 at the age of thirty, sitting for Rossetti to her last day. An overdose of laudanum, taken by accident or with suicidal intent, had finally provided an escape from the lassitude expressed in her gloomy verses.

> Laden autumn, here I stand
> With my sheaves in either hand.
> Speak the word that sets me free,
> Naught but rest seems good to me.

Janet Burden, who became the wife of William Morris, was with Elizabeth Siddal the favorite Pre-Raphaelite model. Although she lived to old age, she, too, was often ill, and went to the Riviera for her health. Judged a ravishing beauty by her contemporaries, she appeared to Henry James as "strange, pale, livid, gaunt, silent, and yet in a manner graceful and picturesque," with "wonderful esthetic hair." When the young G. B. Shaw met her, she looked "at least eight feet high; the effect was as if she had walked out of an Egyptian tomb at Luxor." The Pre-Raphaelite type is largely a combination of Elizabeth's and Janet's features. The fragile silhouette, with long limbs, long fingers, long throat, the tired head leaning on a pillow, with prominent eyes and twisted sensual mouth, became the unhealthy, perverted symbol of Romanticism.[14]

This standard of feminine beauty, certainly created in part by tuberculosis, was accepted with minor modifications all over Europe and North America. The Goncourts describe it with admiration several times in their *Journal*. They refer to the wife of the celebrated chemist, Marcelin Berthelot, as "unforgettable; an intelligent beauty, profound, magnetic, a beauty of soul and of spirit, like one of those unearthly creatures of Edgar Allan Poe . . . great eyes filled with light in the shadow of their rings, the body rather flat beneath a dress that might have been worn by a slender seraphim." Speaking of another woman, they exclaim:

> Looking at those eyes, their contracted pupils as bright in the green light as two black pin heads, those strange, deep, sharp and fascinating eyes, those eyes comparable in their rings to emeralds mounted in fever, I thought how dangerous it would be to meet this woman too often, a danger composed of the immateriality of her person, the supernatural nature of her glance, the emaciation of those features of an almost psychic fineness, that something suprahuman as if belonging to one of Poe's heroines become a Parisian.

Marie Bashkirtsev also accepted disease as contributing to her charm. She noted in her diary: "I cough continually! But for a wonder, far from making me look ugly, this gives me an air of languor that is very becoming."

Less explicit, but no less real, was the effect of phthisis on masculine manners. For instance it probably accounts for the frequent use of high neckwear by the men. A famous Parisian critic, Véron, director of the Opera and sponsor of Rachel, was known to be severely afflicted with scrofula; he always wore a high stock to dissimulate the blemishes caused by the tuberculous glands. This trait led him to be known as "the Prince of Wales" and to receive mail addressed simply to *Monsieur Véron, dans sa cravate, à Paris.*

The wasting and emaciation caused by phthisis added to the glamour of many of the romantic artists and poets just as languor did to the charm of young women. Tom Moore, himself a consumptive, recounts in his diary that he visited Byron, who had been sick in Patras, in February, 1828.

"I look pale," said Byron, looking in the mirror, "I should like to die of a consumption."

"Why?" asked his guest.

"Because the ladies would all say, 'Look at that poor Byron, how interesting he looks in dying!' "

Sidney Lanier, pale, dark, slender and nervous, was the ideal of the bard in the United States. It was consistent with the general attitude that disease and society had thrust upon him that, despite his admiration for Walt Whitman, he was shocked by the healthy animality of that poet's genius.

Sainte-Beuve, who grew to be the fat *bon vivant* shown by his later portraits, nevertheless started his literary life by depicting himself under the name of Joseph Delorme as a pale medical student, suffering from pulmonary phthisis. Even the robust and sensuous Alexandre Dumas made occasional attempts to look frail and consumptive. "In 1823 and 1824," he writes in his memoirs, "it was the fashion to suffer from the lungs; everybody was consumptive, poets especially; it was good form to spit blood after each emotion that was at all sensational, and to die before reaching the age of thirty."

Facetiously Dumas thus alludes to the ancient belief that there exists some relation between tuberculosis and genius. Throughout medical history there runs this suggestion—that the intellectually gifted are the most likely to contract the disease, and furthermore that the same fire which wastes the body in consumption also makes the mind shine with a brighter light. In fact, so much were the Greek physicians impressed with the peculiar nervous force displayed at times by consumptive patients that they invented a word for it. They characterized *spes phthisica* by a perpetual hope of recovery even in the face of devastating disease, and by a feverish urge for accomplishment, as if the patient were anxious to achieve all of which he was potentially capable in an exciting race with death. The Cappadocian Aretæus wrote, in the second century A.D.:

> What is most wonderful is that in a case when blood comes from the lung, in which the disease is most serious, patients do not give up hope. . . . It is simply wonderful how the strength of the body holds out; the strength of the mind even surpasses that of the body.

So many of the famous men and women of the eighteenth and particularly of the nineteenth century were tuberculous—many of them snatching from disease but a few years in which to fulfill their destiny—that the *spes phthisica* came to be generally regarded as favoring intellectual achievement.[15]

"Is it possible that genius is only scrofula?" Elizabeth Barrett Browning overheard someone ask her doctor while she was curing in Torquay. After the discovery of the tubercle bacillus, it appeared logical to postulate the existence of a microbial toxin capable of causing, through a cerebral intoxication, the mental alertness exhibited by so many infected individuals. However, the existence of this toxin and its stimulating effects are purely conjectural.

It is now realized that the classical *spes phthisica* is not as universal a characteristic of tuberculosis as was once thought; but many physicians still believe that there is something peculiar in the psychology of tuberculous patients.[16]

A modern treatise states that the "flickering intelligence which brightens up suddenly for a few hours, but is soon followed by mental depression or fatigue" gives to the consumptive a close resemblance to the person who is under the influence of moderate doses of alcohol, or of a narcotic drug.

> Tuberculous patients, particularly young talented individuals . . . display enormous intellectual capacity of the creative kind. Especially is this to be noted in those who are of the artistic temperament, or who have a talent for imaginative writing. They are in a constant state of nervous irritability, but despite the fact that it hurts their physical condition, they keep on working and produce their best works.[17]

The most extreme manifestation of belief in *spes phthisica* is the statement that the progressive disappearance of tuberculosis is a reason for the decline of literature and the arts in our time. "In the healthful days to come we may not apprehend the past role of tuberculosis in quickening creative faculties; and by way of compensation for good health we may lack certain cultural joys." As creators are often neglected by their contemporaries and honored only by later generations, it is of course impossible to know whether there has been any decline in creative activity, even in the literary and artistic fields. But the feeling that ill-health creates favorable conditions for the finer human attributes is old. Despite their admiration for Victor Hugo, the Goncourts were of the opinion that he would have been an even greater poet had he not been in such robust health. ". . . If a writer is to render the delicacies, the exquisite melancholies, the rare and delicious phantasies, of the vibrant cord of the heart and soul, is it not necessary that he be as Heine was, somewhat crucified personally?"

It is unquestionable that many tuberculous individuals have dazzled the world by the splendor of their emotional and intellectual gifts and by the passionate energy with which they exploited their frail bodies and their few years of life in order to overcome the limitations of disease. Some of them, like Sidney Lanier, have believed that their infirmity was the cause of the consuming restlessness that drove them on to artistic creation. Lanier's disease was punctuated by periods of seeming health, during which he worked with feverish intensity, feeling that his brain was "beating like the heart of haste." "I would think that I am shortly to die, and that my spirit has been singing its swan-song before dissolution. All day my soul hath been cutting swiftly into the great spaces of the subtle, unspeakably deep, driven by wind after wind of heavenly melody."

His exaltation and confidence increased as his malady advanced and his poem "Sunrise" was composed on his deathbed. But like his other works, it lacks that restrained form which is "emotion recollected in tranquility."

John Addington Symonds, also, wrote that tuberculosis had given him a "wonderful Indian summer of experience." He felt that the colors of life had become richer, personal emotions more glowing, perception of intellectual understanding more vivid, and his power over style more masterly during illness, and that he had grown in youth and versatility inversely to his physical decay. But he also knew that he could never summon up sufficient vitality to express what he felt, and he sadly wrote, "I may rave but I shall never rend the heavens. I may sit and sing but I will never make earth listen."

Many consumptive individuals probably display the febrile excitement which made Elizabeth Barrett Browning speak of that "butterfly within, fluttering for release." Katherine Mansfield perceived it in her doctor with the discernment gained from her own personal experience with tuberculosis. "He has the disease himself. I recognize the smile — just the least shade too bright — and his strange joyousness as he came to meet me — the gleam — the faint glitter on the plant that the frost has laid a finger on."

Unfortunately, the consumptive pays a severe penalty for that effervescence, for the excitement of feeling "stingingly alive." It is the sense of frustration that comes from being incapable of expressing in action or even in words the imaginings born of fever. Stevenson wrote "of the baseless ardour, the stimulation of the brain, the sterile joyousness of spirits" that he experienced in the Alps. "It is notable that you are hard to root out of your bed; that you start forth singing, indeed, on your walk, yet are unusually ready to turn home again; that the best of you is volatile; and that although the restlessness remains till night, the strength is early at an end." Keats had experienced this pathetic frustration when he arrived in Naples, so exhausted by disease that he was hardly able to perceive the beauty of the Bay — "Oh! what a misery it is to have an intellect in splints!"

The case of Robert Louis Stevenson is often quoted to support the view that intellectual productivity is increased by active tuberculous disease. But in reality, while it is true that Stevenson wrote some of his best-known works, for example *The Child's Garden of Verses, The Strange Case of Dr. Jekyll and Mr. Hyde, Kidnapped,* when he was almost physically disabled by tuberculosis, he also did much creative writing during his periods of good health. All accounts of his sojourn in the South Seas bear witness to the gusto with which he enjoyed his new life.

> It is like a fairy-story that I should have recovered liberty and strength, and should go round again among my fellow-men, boating, riding, bathing, toiling hard with a wood-knife in the forest. . . .

> This climate; these landfalls at dawn; new islands peeking from the morning bank; new forested harbours; new passing alarms of squalls and surf, new interests of gentle natives — the whole tale of my life is better to me than any poem.

And yet, in the midst of all these happy activities, he wrote during the last three years of his life several novels considered among his greatest writing.[18]

There may be, nevertheless, some basis for the statement that consumption fosters and nourishes genius. Within certain limits fever from any source can heighten emotion, sharpen perception and render intellectual processes more lucid and rapid. "Six weeks with fever is an eternity," wrote Balzac. "Hours are like days . . . then the nights are not lost."

Since consumptives often experience mild fever without gross toxemia and without physical prostration, they may crave a full life and exhibit eagerness to seize the fleeting moments for creative efforts. Furthermore, the decreased physical vigor of the tuberculous patient limits his ability to fulfill natural urges and thereby increases his tendency to sublimate them into those forms of mental activity that are most natural to him. "Those who would imagine must not live," wrote the Goncourts.[19] For most sensitive temperaments, artistic expression is a kind of bloodletting, and Symonds spoke endlessly of the relief from his miseries that he found through writing.

Accounts of the medical treatment of phthisis during the nineteenth century reveal that opiates were then almost universally used to quiet cough and diarrhea, and to ease mental anguish. Opium-eating had been adopted by the Romantics in the circle of Schilling in Germany, then also in England and France. It had become part of an esthetic creed, a means of liberating the unconscious, of achieving unity with Nature and release from the constraints of society.

Many writers were aware of the strange quality that opiates gave to their thoughts. "Opium," said De Quincey, "gives and takes away. It defeats the steady habit of exertion; but it creates spasms of irregular exertion! It ruins the natural power of life; but it develops preternatural paroxysms of intermitting power."

Coleridge probably owed some of his abnormal brain-states to the use of opium. The drug had been prescribed for him at school when he was suffering from rheumatic fever and he had often resorted to it later to relieve insomnia and to allay pain. "Laudanum gave me repose, not sleep," he wrote to his brother; "but you, I believe, know how divine this repose is, what a spot of enchantment, a green spot of fountain and flowers and trees in the very heart of a waste of sands." According to Coleridge's own account, he wrote "Kubla Khan" without any effort upon waking from a dream under the influence of opium.

It is probable that every consumptive became, in some measure, an opium addict, and it may be wondered whether the drug did not contribute to the mental effervescence that expressed itself in poetry and artistic creation. Needless to say, it is only in those endowed with genius and already possessed of the creative urge that opium facilitates literary expression, and De Quincey's remark in regard to the opium addict is equally true of the tuberculous patient: "If a man 'whose talk is of oxen' should become an opium-eater, the probability is that (if he is not too dull to dream at all) — he will dream about oxen."

Even granted that tuberculosis can under certain circumstances stimulate spasms of creative eagerness, it is all too certain that the cost is often greater than the achievement, for periods of overactivity usually bring about extension of the disease as their sequel. The more eager and imaginative the patient, the more willingly he grasps at any stimulating influence — and, as a result, the more difficulty he has in checking the progress of his disease.

There is no evidence that tuberculosis breeds genius. The

probability is, rather, that eagerness for achievement often leads to a way of life that renders the body less resistant to infection.

In *A Study of British Genius* Havelock Ellis emphasized that tuberculosis was present in at least forty distinguished Britishers of the nineteenth century. To present a fair view of the case, he should have mentioned also examples that belie the alleged relation between tuberculosis and genius. For instance, of the six children of Thomas Anthony Trollope, four died of tuberculosis between the ages of twelve and thirty-three, without giving any evidence of creative ability.[20] The literary fame of the family rests on the mother and the two other children, Thomas Adolphus and Anthony, who enjoyed robust health throughout their lives. At a period when one fourth of the deaths were due to tuberculosis, and when exposure to infection was well-nigh universal, it is not surprising to find that many creative individuals also died or suffered from the disease. The wonder is that many more did not become consumptive, and were allowed to enjoy long and healthy years of productivity!

The attitude of perverted sentimentalism toward tuberculosis began to change in the last third of the nineteenth century. In reaction against the artificialities of the Romantic Era, writers and artists rediscovered that disease was not necessarily poetical, and health not detrimental to creative power. Turning their eyes away from the languorous, fainting young women and their romantic lovers, they noticed instead the miserable humanity living in the dreary tenements born of the Industrial Revolution. In the "tentacular cities" they saw hosts of men, women and children, pale too, often cold and starving, working long hours in dark and crowded shops, breathing smoke and coal dust. Tuberculosis was there, breeding suffering and misery without romance. And, little by little, it dawned on social common sense what a mockery it was to depict consumption as a spiritualization of the being, as a romantic experience detached from the horrid aspects of disease. In the laboring classes consumption was not the aristocratic decline, inspiring works of art and leading painlessly to an ethereal release of the soul among the falling autumn leaves. It was the great killer and breeder of destitution. The writers of the realist school, who visited slums and hospitals that they might observe the sick and the poor, acknowledged in dark words the bodies distorted by cough, the faces livid with asphyxiation, the minds haunted by the thought of death.[21]

The germ theory caused a still further evolution in the attitude toward disease, detectable both in literature and in the reaction of the general public. Consumption had been exploited by the Victorian novelist as the manifestation of an inexorable fate that won for the hero the sympathy of the reader. But tuberculosis now became a contagion, something unclean.[22] In several modern novels, the infected individual became almost an untouchable, a character stimulating repulsion or fear.

Consumption, which had been for half a century the muse of literature, became a blot on society, the symbol of all that was rotten in the industrial world. Against it, in a great crusade for health, turned the champions of a happier, more smiling life.

Part Two

THE CAUSES OF TUBERCULOSIS

CHAPTER VI

Phthisis, Consumption and Tubercles

In 1881 August Flint published in collaboration with William H. Welch the fifth edition of his standard textbook *The Principles and Practice of Medicine.* The authors dealt at length with the subject of tuberculosis, mentioning as its causes: hereditary disposition, unfavorable climate, sedentary indoor life, defective ventilation, deficiency of light and "depressing emotions." They added that "the doctrine of the contagiousness of the disease has . . . its advocates, but general belief is in its non-communicability."[1] Never did a textbook statement become so soon and so completely outmoded, for it was the following year, in 1882, that Robert Koch published his epoch-making paper announcing the discovery of tubercle bacilli and demonstrating that they are the primary cause of the disease.

After Koch, it became easy to recognize that the different forms of tuberculosis in the various organs of the body all possess one element in common, namely the damage caused by the bacilli multiplying in the infected tissues. But before this unifying concept became available, the physician was faced with a confusing array of signs and symptoms, bearing no obvious relation one to the other. The sharper his clinical acumen and the wider his experience, the more skilled he became in differentiating these signs and symptoms, and the greater was his tendency to regard them as the expression of different maladies. Hence the countless names under which the various types of tuberculous infections have been described in the past; hence also the many theories that have been devised to account for their genesis and evolution.

We shall recount in the following pages how a few physicians succeeded in organizing this welter of information into an orderly system based purely on clinical and pathological criteria, long before the discovery of the tubercle bacillus. We shall note also that much theoretical and practical knowledge was gathered by those who regarded heredity, nutrition, climate, or emotions as the causes of tuberculosis. The progressive discovery of facts, and the unfolding of doctrines bearing on the causation of tuberculosis, constitute some of the most brilliant chapters in the history of medical science. They demonstrate that a disease can be described and analyzed in terms of many unrelated theories, each true at its own level, each fruitful in understanding and practical results. To him who follows her way, Nature reveals many roads that lead in the direction of truth.

Ancient knowledge of disease was derived almost exclusively from the observation of symptoms. As the initial stages of tuberculosis cause little discomfort, and usually remain unnoticed by the patient, the disease came under medical attention only in its very advanced form until modern times. Hippocrates, who lived about 400 B.C., and most physicians until the nineteenth century, taught that phthisis begins as a respiratory catarrh, with chest pains, increasing malaise and a dry cough yielding yellow sputum; but it is now known that, in many cases, these symptoms occur only after the lesions have become extensive. The Greek and Roman physicians recognized that evening fever and night sweats, blood spitting, a small pulse, clubbed fingers and curved nails, pleurisy followed by empyema, extinction of voice and diarrhea, were signs often associated with pulmonary phthisis. However, what impressed them most was the emaciation of the patient, an exhaustion of the reserves of the body that they traced to the "vehement" or "hectic" fever characteristic of the disease.

"Phthoe" was the name given by the Greeks to the individual shriveling up under intense heat; and the word "phthisis" eventually came to designate the wasting and melting away of the body caused by disease of the lungs. The Cappadocian monk Aretæus, a Greek practicing medicine in Asia Minor, wrote around 200 B.C. a description of the phthisical patient that has become classical:

> Voice hoarse; neck slightly bent, tender, not flexible, somewhat extended; fingers slender but joints thick; of the bones alone the figure remains, for the fleshy parts are wasted; the nails of the fingers crooked, their pulps are shriveled and flat, for, owing to the loss of flesh, they neither retain their tension nor rotundity; and owing to the same cause, the nails are bent, namely, because it is the compact flesh at their points which is intended as a support to them; and the tension thereof is like that of solids. Nose sharp, slender; cheeks prominent and red; eyes hollow, brilliant and glittering; swollen, pale, or livid in the countenance; the slender parts of the jaws rest upon the teeth, as if smiling; otherwise of a cadaverous aspect. So also in all other respects; slender, without flesh; the muscles of the arms imperceptible; not a vestige of the mammae, the nipples only to be seen; one may not only count the ribs themselves, but also easily trace them to their terminations; for even the articulations at the vertebrae are quite visible and their connections with the sternum are also manifest; the intercostal spaces are hollow and rhomboidal, agreeably to the configuration of the bone; hypochondriac region lank and retracted; the abdomen and flanks contiguous to the spine. Joints clearly developed, prominent, devoid of flesh, so also with the tibia, ischium, and the humerus; the spine of the vertebrae, formerly hollow, now protrudes, the muscles on either side being wasted; the whole shoulder blades apparent like wings of birds.

The Latin word *tabes,* used in a general sense to denote wasting, was applied more specifically to phthisis by Fracastorius in the seventeenth century. We have seen that its translation as "decline" found great favor in the early nineteenth century. Words expressing the emaciation of tuberculous patients occur in all languages, but probably none has been more widely used than "consumption." To describe the process that caused their patients to burn up with fever and lose weight, the English physicians of the early seventeenth century adopted the Latin verb *consumere,* meaning to eat up or devour; later they formed the habit of referring to wasting diseases as "a consumption" when it became proper to discuss medical problems in the vernacular. Diseases other than pulmonary phthisis which can cause wasting of the body – diabetes, cancer, abscesses of the lungs caused by a variety of microorganisms – are also described as "a consumption" in literature of the eighteenth century. The common meaning of the word is defined as follows by Benjamin Marten in the first chapter of his book, *A New Theory of Consumption, more especially of a Phthisis or Consumption of the Lungs,* published in 1722 in London:

> Custom has now so much prevailed with Physicians that whenever they speak of a Consumption it is generally and more especially taken for a Phthisis or that Consumption of the Body which has its rise from an Ulceration of the Lungs.
>
> A Phthisis or Consumption of the Lungs may be very justly defined to be a wearing away or consuming of all the muscular or fleshy Parts of the Body, accompanied with a Cough, purulent Spitting, hectic Fever, shortness of Breath, Night Sweats, etc.

The anatomo-pathological era began with the Renaissance. Dissatisfied with vague explanations of disease based on the observation of fever, aches and wasting, physicians started to search for more concrete knowledge by dissecting the bodies of dead patients. They felt confident that the anatomical alterations found at autopsy would help them to determine the primary seat and cause of illness, and indeed, they soon discovered that the wasting of phthisis was constantly associated with the presence of curious lesions in the inner organs. In the first half of the sixteenth century, Jean Fernel described the cavities of the phthisical lung under the name of "vomicae." In 1679, Franciscus Delaboe Sylvius reported in his *Opera Medica* that he had found particularly in the lungs, but also in other parts of the body, characteristic nodules that he called "tubercles," which were wont to suppurate and give rise to "ulcers." While performing an autopsy on a youth in 1700, Manget observed tubercles so small as to resemble "millet seed" present in all parts of the body, lungs, spleen, mesentery, intestine. It is to commemorate Manget's description that this type of disseminated disease is now called "miliary" tuberculosis.

As observations increased, it became obvious that the tubercles, ulcers and cavities could occur in all sizes and exhibit many varied characteristics. Tubercles could be hard as cartilage, as bone, or even appear to be made of chalk. In other cases they contained puslike material of different degrees of softness — "like suet or like honey." About 1790 Matthew Baillie described in certain tubercles an unusual type of "cheeselike" material, the now familiar "caseous" matter. It was known also that, in addition to the sharply limited tubercles and cavities, there often occurred in phthisical lungs ill-defined areas of inflammation, more extensively described later under the name of "infiltration."

Thus, an enormous volume of precise and detailed anatomical knowledge accumulated through the seventeenth and eighteenth centuries, but mere description of these findings did not satisfy the speculative mind. How did all these peculiar lesions arise in the lung and in the other organs, and what relation did they bear to phthisis? Many physicians thought that tubercles were, in reality, nothing but minute glands normally present in the tissues but damaged and enlarged by disease, whereas others held that they were entirely new structures arising *de novo* in the midst of normal tissues, like a kind of tumor. There were endless speculations to account for the many puzzling facts revealed by anatomical studies. How did it come about that tubercles could be either chalky or bonelike, full of pus or cheesy? What determined the size of the cavities and the raw or spongy or smooth character of their surface? Why did some remain closed, and others present an opening into bronchi or blood vessels? Did the tubercles occurring in parts of the body other than the lungs bear any relation to pulmonary phthisis — for example, were the swollen lymph nodes that disfigured the neck of scrofulous patients related in any way to the lesions found in the chest? Most physicians were inclined to regard these diverse pathological manifestations as signs of unrelated diseases, and they tried to bring some order into the confused mass of anatomical knowledge by carefully separating one from the other and classifying the conditions characterized by different types of tubercles, ulcers and cavities.

Every system of classification suggested a new theory of the nature of pulmonary phthisis. Although little has survived of these pioneering attempts at formulating a rational explanation of disease, it seems worth outlining their general trends, were it only to illustrate the blundering way in which the collective human mind slowly progresses toward truth.

It had long been held that phthisis could be the outcome of nonspecific forms of chest ailments caused by many types of irritation: persistent colds with material draining from the sinuses into the lungs, excessive coughing, blood spitting, reaction to toxic material present in the air, and other causes. Said Thomas Willis in his *Practise of Physick*, published in 1684, "In the lungs rather than in the Heart or Brain the threads of Life are and there they are oftenest broken"; phthisis is "a withering away of the body from an ill formation of the Lungs." In his monumental *Phthisiologia*, Richard Morton presented in 1689 what appeared to him a complete picture and theory of phthisis. Like others, he did point to the causative role of all sorts of nonspecific irritating effects and claimed furthermore that the tubercles often originated from a "stuffing of the lung with serum" due to some defect in circulation of the blood.[2] He was inclined to believe that all types of tubercular nodes found in the body, those of scrofula in particular, had a similar origin and therefore did bear some relation to phthisis.[3] He traced the fever and other symptoms of consumption to a tendency of the tubercles to "ripen" and turn into abscesses or cavities. "For in the lungs of the dead body we found at the same time some tubercles that were turned to 'aposthemes' and others that were inflamed; and lastly, some that were crude and unripe."[4] Morton also stressed that the course of disease is influenced by many general factors, such as natural constitution, food, physical rest, peace of mind. The effect of age, for example, he illustrated by the following statement, "The consumption of young men, that are in the flower of their age, when the heat of the blood is yet brisk, and therefore more disposed to a feverish fermentation, is for the most part acute. But in old men, where the natural heat is decayed, it is more chronical."

Mixed with the shrewd observations described by the old physicians in their quaint language, one finds many wordy and puerile attempts to give a logical account of the genesis of tuberculosis. These dreary pages of antiquated theory appear, at first, as so much uncritical and wasted effort. And yet, it is out of the welter of their confused arguments that there slowly emerged the modern technique of medical research. This technique, which yielded such spectacular advances in the understanding of disease during the early part of the nineteenth century, depends in essence on the integration of pathological and of clinical observations. The careful practice of post-mortem examinations first led to the study of the extreme, terminal forms of lesions in each type of disease, then to the detection of less obvious tissue changes. This anatomical knowledge served as a basis for the formulation of hypotheses concerning the evolution of each disease from its early phase to its ultimate manifestations. On the other hand, by correlating the type of lesions found after death with the signs and symptoms recognized during the life of the patient, physicians learned to interpret their clinical findings in terms of organic alterations and to classify diseases on the basis of combined clinical and pathological observations.

This dual approach to medical research made even more acute the need for precise and objective methods to examine, in the living body, the seat and extent of the disease process. From time immemorial, methods of physical examination had been limited to a crude measurement of the temperature and pulse, and to a sketchy practice of palpation. Now and then, the physician went so far as to apply his ear to the body of the patient in order to detect some abnormal sound, but on the whole, he depended upon cough, fever and wasting to diagnose pulmonary diseases.

Examination of the chest became possible only after the discovery of percussion by Auenbrugger in 1761 and of mediate auscultation with the stethoscope by Laënnec in 1816. So simple in principle are these two techniques, so completely independent of complex theoretical knowledge, that one may well wonder why they had not been discovered and practiced much earlier. As we shall see, percussion and mediate auscultation were invented by two busy clinicians who had certainly felt the need of recognizing in their patients during life the lesions which they suspected to be present on the basis of experience derived from post-mortem studies. In medicine, as in other endeavors, necessity is often the mother of invention.

CHAPTER VII

Percussion, Auscultation and the Unitarian Theory of Phthisis

LEOPOLD VON AUENBRUGGER was born in 1722 in the Austrian city of Graz, the son of an innkeeper and of a mother who was much interested in music. As a youth he certainly had many occasions to watch his father determine the fluid remaining in beer and wine barrels by tapping their sides; and his mother's influence must have educated his ear to recognize subtle differences in sounds and tones. In later life he wrote a comic opera, *The Chimney Sweep*, that was played at the Court in Vienna, but he had found long before a more original application of his musical background in the field of medicine.

After becoming a physician Auenbrugger described in his *Inventum novum*, published in 1761, a new method for the detection of diseases of the chest. The method was based on the observation that the thorax, on being tapped, yields in different locations characteristic voices that become modified in disease, "higher, deeper, clearer, more obscure or almost suffocated." He observed that "the sound elicited from a healthy chest resembles the stifled sound of a drum covered with a thick woolen cloth." With much care and love of precise detail, he learned to interpret the tones derived by striking the chest with the massed tips of the fingers, advising that the skin of the chest be covered with a tight shirt or the fingers gloved with unpolished leather so as to minimize noises that would interfere with the natural sounds.

He recognized that "if a place naturally sonorous and now sounding only as a piece of board when struck still retains the same sound, on percussion, when the breath is held after a deep inspiration, we must conclude that the disease extends deep into the cavity of the chest." He described the different sounds heard over lung cavities, either filled with fluids or empty. Discussing empyema, he noticed the increased sound above the area of dullness when the fluid fills only part of the thorax and the changes in location of the sound by modifying the position of the patient. "If the chest is only half filled, a louder sound will be obtained over the parts to which the fluid does not extend; and, in this case, the resonance will be found to vary according to the position of the patient and the consequent level which the fluid attains."

The technique of percussion made it easy to do what had been thought impossible, namely to perceive during life some of the alterations with which pathologists had become familiar at the autopsy table. Auenbrugger was ennobled in 1784 and became a popular character at the Court in Vienna, but despite this personal success, little heed was paid to his *Inventum novum.* For all intents and purposes, percussion was forgotten until rediscovered by Corvisard some thirty years later.

It had taken a physician with an educated ear and a creative imagination to discover percussion, but it took one with a dynamic personality to make the world aware of its usefulness. Jean Nicolas Corvisard was born in 1755. He studied medicine in Paris. Accepted to practice at the Hôpital Necker, he was instructed to wear a wig while attending at the hospital, but with the vigor that characterized his behavior throughout life, he refused to submit with the remark that "respect for outward signs must not degenerate into superstition." Notwithstanding this display of independence, he advanced rapidly in the Paris medical world and became in 1797 Professor of Medicine at the

Collège de France. Napoleon, who had no faith in medicine but great faith in Corvisard and respected his independent spirit, appointed him his Physician in Ordinary.

It was in 1797 that Corvisard read in an obscure treatise an account of Auenbrugger's technique of percussion. After having convinced himself of its practical usefulness in diagnostic work and of the ease with which it could be used at the bedside, he undertook to translate Auenbrugger's book to make it available to his French students and colleagues. This translation exerted a far-reaching influence by helping to mold the point of view of the Paris clinical school. For Corvisard was no ordinary teacher. Perhaps the first in the history of medicine, he stressed with equal forcefulness the need for thorough physical examination of the patient at the bedside and the importance of elaborate autopsy work. The decisive influence of this teaching is epitomized in three of his pupils: Dupuytren, who was to rule over French surgery for half a century, Bayle and Laënnec, who left an indelible stamp on internal medicine and revolutionized, in particular, the knowledge of tuberculosis.

Gaspard Laurent Bayle, born in 1774, became assistant in anatomy to Corvisard in 1802 and was appointed to the medical staff of the Hôpital de la Charité in 1805. Austere and exacting to the highest degree, in his moral convictions as well as in his work, he was, according to Laënnec, "gifted with wondrous powers of concentration and perseverance; nothing could tire or dishearten him, indeed application seemed to be so inherent in his habits that none of his friends and fellow-workers ever saw him, through lassitude, discouragement or neglect, omit to do that which was to be done."

The indefatigable Bayle recorded the detailed histories of all the individual cases of illness that occurred in his hospital service, writing down in his notebooks not only his prognosis, but also his anticipation of the organic changes to be found after death. Within a few years, he performed some nine hundred autopsies, comparing in each case his anticipation with the actual findings. The comparative study of his clinical and pathological observations led him to a number of conclusions that have stood the test of time and he showed, in particular, that a small tubercle was the starting point of many of the lesions of phthisis. He recognized that the complications observed in the larynx, intestine and lymph nodes were further manifestations of the same disease, and he stated that the cheesy matter found in tubercles was a characteristic production of phthisis. Unimpeachable in his objective findings, Bayle lacked the inspired vision that would have permitted him to integrate his observations into a single theory. Noting that tubercles were found not only in the lungs, but also in other parts of the body of consumptives, he postulated, as had everybody before him, that consumption was the result of some obscure general defect of the body, a "dyscrasia" or "diathesis," words as vague as the thought that they were trying to express. Failing to recognize any unifying character in the clinical history of his patients and in the material derived from his autopsies, he laboriously and wrongly concluded that the cases of wasting due to lung conditions studied by him could be divided into six different diseases, only one of which he regarded as true tuberculous phthisis.

In 1816, at the age of forty-two, Bayle died of tuberculosis, leaving an immense monument of useful labor. A few years before his death he had heard his younger friend Laënnec proclaim with the inspired assurance of genius the unitarian theory of phthisis.

René Théophile Hyacinthe Laënnec was born in French Brittany in 1781.[1] His mother died young, when he was only six years old, at the confinement of her fourth child, who died shortly after. It is certain that her three brothers also died young, and it has been suggested that she was consumptive. More or less abandoned by their charming but irresponsible father, Laënnec and his brother Michaud went in 1787 to live for one year with one of their uncles, rector of a parish nearby, who died a few years later of consumption. In 1788, the two boys were sent to their other uncle, who practiced and taught medicine in Nantes. There – in October, 1795 – Laënnec entered the medical school at the age of fourteen years and seven months.

These were strenuous times for the boy. Long walks in the country, hunting, the collecting of minerals, plants, insects and birds' eggs, the raising of rabbits, a thorough study of Greek, Latin and English were activities which competed, but did not interfere, with his medical curriculum. His pride hurt by poverty and by the lack of suitable clothes, he decided to overcome his social handicap by mastering music, poetry, drawing and dancing. He developed a passion for playing the flute that never abandoned him, and his skill as a draughtsman survives in an extraordinary self-portrait that he sketched and lithographed himself later in life (around 1820). Life continued as intense physically as mentally all through his stay in Nantes. "Each moment that I lose seems to me a century," once wrote the eager boy. In 1789 he developed a high fever, with great prostration, nose bleed and, for a time, pain in the chest, probably the first overt signs of the tuberculous disease that was to kill him later. He soon recovered and devoted his convalescence to playing the flute.

In 1799 more excitement came into his life when he was enlisted in the medical corps of the National Guard to participate in the civil war against the Chouans. He returned to Nantes after several months of service, and, having finally received a small stipend from his father, set out by carriage for Paris, there to complete his medical training. Ignoring a febrile cold, he decided to walk the last two hundred miles of the trip from Angers to the capital. Ten days later in May, 1801, he took quarters with his brother, Michaud, then a student in Paris. Michaud died of tuberculosis nine years later after beginning with brilliance a career in the law.

Life in Paris proved even more strenuous than in Nantes. At the Hôpital de la Charité, Laënnec followed the course of the stern Corvisard, whose aphorisms he carefully wrote down and published later. He attended the lectures in pathological anatomy delivered by Bichat, who died of tuberculosis the following year at the age of thirty-one. He did special work under Bayle and Dupuytren, performing with them dissections, again dissections, and still more dissections. During his first three years at the Charité, he drew up a minute history of nearly four hundred patients. All these studies went on despite ill health and lack of funds. In his poor lodgings he would sit writing at his desk, naked to the waist to overcome the discomfort of profuse sweating. More and more he came to suffer from bad spells of asthma and dyspnea, intestinal ailments and continuous headaches. Many a time he infected his fingers in the course of dissection, but clinical work and autopsies went on uninterrupted. He found time, in addition, to write as his thesis for the doctorate a treatise on Hippocrates based on a study of the master's writings in the original Greek. He taught private students, edited medical journals, engaged in lively controversies, and contributed original investigations to the scientific literature.

For distraction he returned now and then to his early interest in natural history and perfected himself in English. He became proficient in the Celtic dialect and in the folklore of his native Brittany. This permitted him in 1814 to organize special wards in Paris for the care of the wounded Breton soldiers who did not comprehend French and with whom he conversed in their native tongue. When too ill to work, he found relief in long walks and hunting. Away from Paris on vacation with friends, his fanciful spirit would again find expression in verse, music, playwriting and songs. Back in Brittany he became interested in farming and all aspects of country life.

An authentic account describes him as only five feet, three inches tall. But despite this small stature, he appeared too high for his frame, thin as a shadow as he was. The complexion was blemished, the eyes sunken; he had prominent cheekbones and hollow cheeks, his weasel face was emaciated. His nose and lips were thin, his blue-gray eyes calm and reflective, but his dynamic bearing and his enthusiasm inspired in his associates and patients the utmost devotion. The painting of him by Alexandre Dubois and the pen sketch that he made of himself agree well with this description. It is against this background of poor health, and of many-sided interests pursued with lustful intensity, that we must briefly review the phenomenal scientific achievements crowded by this small, asthmatic, dry, emaciated Breton into the few years of his tormented life.

Shortly after his arrival in Paris, Laënnec began under Bayle's influence anatomical and clinical researches on the problem of phthisis. Supplementing the work of his instructor, with whom he established a close and lasting friendship, he was in a position to announce in 1803 that they had found tubercles in all organs of the body, muscle and bone included. The diversity in structure of the tubercles and the presence in the phthisical lung of many types of ulcers and cavities made it appear at the time that a multiplicity of different diseases were encompassed under the word "phthisis." William Stark, in England, had held a contrary opinion a few decades earlier, claiming that ordinary lung tubercles could evolve into ulcers and possibly into cavities, thus suggesting in fact that these lesions were different manifestations of the same disease. But Stark had died at the age of twenty-nine; and his observations, based on only ten autopsies, were largely ignored and without any influence on medical thinking.

Despite his close association and intimate friendship with Bayle, who taught that phthisis corresponded to at least six independent diseases, Laënnec soon became convinced that the various lesions found in the phthisical lung were, in reality, all different phases in the evolution of the same pathological process. With incredible energy, he proceeded to trace pulmonary phthisis through all its manifestations in over two hundred cadavers, from the tiniest gray tubercle, through the masses of cheesy material, to the cavities in all their aspects. As a result of these studies, he was soon in a position to state that "Whatever be the form under which the tuberculous matter is developed, it presents at first the appearance of a gray semitransparent substance which gradually acquires a fluidity nearly equal to that of pus. When the softened material is expelled through the bronchi, cavities are left, commonly known under the name of ulcers of the lungs, but which I shall designate tuberculous excavations." Without the help of the microscope, ignorant of the tubercle bacillus, he also recognized that "the matter of tubercles can arise in the lungs or in other organs, either as separated, well-defined structures, or as interstitial injection or infiltration."

It was in March, 1804, less than three years after his arrival in Paris and after the beginning of his researches, that Laënnec delivered the famous lecture in which he set forth his revolutionary views on the genesis of pulmonary phthisis, stating in brief that infiltration, tubercles and cavities were the expression of a single disease and that the different forms of phthisis were merely different aspects of tuberculosis of the lung. In 1839, J. L. Schönlein, Professor of Medicine in Zürich, suggested that the word "tuberculosis" be used as a generic name for all the manifestations of phthisis, since the tubercle was the fundamental anatomical basis of the disease. Thus, three years of work by the young, emaciated, consumptive Laënnec had brought an unexpected solution to a debate that had lasted for more than twenty centuries.

Laënnec devoted the following decade of his life to the further development of his thoughts on tuberculosis and contributed many other important facts to various fields of clinical medicine.

By 1816, he was widely recognized as a master of morbid anatomy and as a polished clinician. When Bayle died, he was designated to replace him as medical officer to the Hôpital Necker. It was shortly thereafter that he devised mediate auscultation by means of the stethoscope, a technique that revolutionized the art of physical examination.

Auscultation, of course, was not entirely new. Hippocrates had mentioned in *De Morbis* that the gurgling sound of death rattle can be heard as "a slight noise like the boiling of vinegar" by holding the ear close to the side of the thorax. He had described also that a "noise like that of rubbing against a leather strap" could be heard in cases of pleuritis. These hints probably did not escape Laënnec during his early study of the Greek master. The surgeon Ambroise Paré had described in the sixteenth century the clicks and clocks due to reductions of dislocation, and had noticed some of the chest sounds, "If there is slush . . . in the thorax, one hears a sound as of a bottle half full which gurgles."

At the beginning of the eighteenth century Robert Hooke had prophesied the "possibility of discovering the internal motions and actions of the bodies by the sound they make."

> Who knows but that, as in a watch, we may hear the beating of the balance, and the running of the wheels, and the striking of the hammers, and the grating of the teeth and multitudes of other noises — who knows, I say, but that it may be possible to discover the motions of the internal parts of bodies, whether animal, vegetable or mineral, by the sound they make; that one may discover the works performed in the several offices and shops of a man's body and thereby discover what instrument or engine is out of order, what works are going on at several times and lie still at others and the like. . . . I have been able to hear very plainly the beating of a man's heart; and it is common to hear the motion of the wind to and fro in the guts and other small vessels; the stopping in the lungs is easily dis-

> covered by the wheezing, the stopping of the head by the humming and whistling noises, the slipping to and fro of the joints, in many cases by crackling and the like.

Although *direct* auscultation had thus long been known to be theoretically possible, it was little practiced; Laënnec himself felt that, "exclusive of reason of decorum" it was impracticable in obese individuals or in the female over the space occupied by the mammae. Furthermore, he objected to the method because of the frequent occurrence of vermin on the bodies of patients. But eager as he was to understand the evolution of disease processes, he felt acutely the need of techniques that would help him to detect during life the nature and extent of organic lesions. It was with this problem in mind that he witnessed one day in the garden of the Louvre a spectacle that inspired him to invent *mediate* auscultation. Two groups of youngsters were playing at either end of a long beam of wood. One of them would scratch the end of the log with a pin, while the others, setting their ears against the wood at the other end, would hoot with joy when they heard the scratch clearly transmitted through the solid medium.

Laënnec had, at the Hôpital Necker, a young woman patient whose heart he was anxious to examine and the game which he had just witnessed gave him an idea. Arrived at the hospital, he took a calling card, rolled it up tightly and tied it. Placing this improvised instrument upon the heart area, he found that the sounds came to his ear much more clearly than he had ever heard them before! It was somewhat later that he coined the term "stethoscope" for his new instrument, by combining two Greek words meaning "the chest" and "to examine."

With his usual driving energy, Laënnec immediately began to improve the stethoscope, himself turning on a lathe several types of hollow rods made of various kinds of wood. Exploring with it the vast clinical material available on his hospital service, he reached within a few months an incredible degree of skill in the technique of mediate auscultation. He read his preliminary paper on auscultation before the Academy of Sciences in February 1818, and in 1819 described at length his finding in a larger treatise, *De L'Auscultation Médiate ou Traité du Diagnostic des Maladies des Poumons et du Cœur fondé Principalement sur ce Nouveau Moyen d'Exploration.* In the first part of the book Laënnec presents the plan of his clinical studies.

> I shall divide my work into four parts. The first will deal with the signs that can be obtained from the voice when heard by means of the cylinder [stethoscope]; the second with those furnished by the respiratory sounds; the third with those supplied by *râles;* and, by way of appendix, the results at which I have arrived in my investigations on the effusion of liquids into the various cavities of the thorax; the fourth will contain an analysis of the heartbeats in health and in sickness, and an account of the special signs characterizing diseases of the heart and aorta.

Laënnec gave precise and original descriptions of clinical symptoms and post-mortem appearances of pulmonary tuberculosis, pneumonia, pulmonary edema, pulmonary gangrene, emphysema, dilation of the bronchial tubes, hydrothorax, pneumothorax and some forms of cardiac disease. He showed that it was possible to predict by mediate auscultation what would be found after death and elaborated on his demonstration that all phthisis is tuberculous. His descriptions of chest and heart sounds have become famous in medical literature. He used the term *râle* to express all the sounds caused by "the passage of the air through the fluids of bronchia or lungs or by its transmission through any of the air passages partially contracted." And he added, "These sounds likewise accompany the cough and are made even more perceptible by it." The term *râle,* referring in French to "death rattle," was objectionable to patients, and Laënnec used instead the Latin *rhonchus,* meaning a "snort" or "frog croak." To illustrate his style and method of work, it seems worth quoting his description of the discovery of pectoriloquy, the peculiar sound detected with the stethoscope over pulmonary cavities.

> In the very earliest period of my researches on mediate auscultation I attempted to ascertain the differences which the sound of the voice might cause within the chest. In examining several subjects with this in view I was struck by the discovery of a very singular phenomenon. I was studying the case of a woman affected with a slight bilious fever and a cough having the character of a pulmonary catarrh. When I applied the cylinder below the middle of the right clavicle while she was speaking, her voice appeared to come directly from the chest and to reach the ear through the central canal of the instrument. This peculiar phenomenon was confined to a space about an inch square and was not detectable in any other part of the chest. In order to elucidate the cause of this singularity I examined most of the patients in the hospital and recognized the same phenomenon in about twenty of them. . . . The subsequent death in the hospital of many of the individuals who had exhibited it enabled me to ascertain the correctness of my suppositions; in every case I found in the lungs excavations of various sizes, resulting from the dissolution of tubercles, and all communicating with the bronchi by openings of different diameters. . . . This circumstance naturally led me to think that pectoriloquy is caused by the superior vibration produced by the voice in parts having a more solid and wider extent of surface, and I imagined that, if this were so, the same effect ought to result from the application of the cylinder to the larynx and trachea of a person in health. My conjecture proved correct.

In principle and practice, the method of mediate auscultation is as simple as the method of percussion. And yet the invention of the stethoscope was at first received with as much indifference as was Auenbrugger's discovery. One of the only laudatory accounts was written by Chateaubriand, in reviewing some of the important events of the year; but the writer's interest probably came from the fact that he and his wife were Laënnec's patients.

Even those who professed great admiration for Laënnec's medical genius and were intrigued by his stethoscope regarded the instrument as merely a mechanical toy, out of place in the proud and dignified art of medicine. For example Forbes, who wrote the first English translation of the treatise on mediate auscultation, expressed a somewhat scornful skepticism in his preface.

> That it will ever come into general use notwithstanding its value, I am extremely doubtful; because its beneficial application requires much time and gives a good deal of trouble both to the patient and the practitioner; because its whole hue and character are foreign, and opposed to all our habits and associations. It must be confessed that there is something even ludicrous in the picture of a grave physician proudly listening through a long tube applied to the patient's thorax, as if the disease were a living being that could communicate its condition to the sense without. Besides, there is in this method a sort of bold claim and pretension to certainty and precision in diagnosis, which cannot at first sight but be somewhat startling to a mind deeply versed in the knowledge and uncertainties of our art, and to the calm and cautious habits of philosophizing to which the English physician is accustomed.[2]

But Laënnec was not one to be readily discouraged. To his cousin, Meriadec, who was preparing a thesis on auscultation, he wrote, "Do not fear to repeat what has already been said. Men need these things dinned into their ears many times and from all sides. The first rumor makes them prick up their ears, the second registers and the third enters." After a few years the celebrated French physician, Pierre Louis, introduced the stethoscope in his service at the Hôpital de la Charité in Paris. And before long the "Stethoscope Song," a sketch written by Oliver Wendell Holmes of Boston, served as a symbol of international recognition.[3] Within a decade mediate auscultation came to be recognized as the most valuable of the diagnostic tools. Along with percussion it remained for a whole century, until the discovery of X rays, the only method available for the physical examination of the chest. Thanks to it, the knowledge derived from studies at the autopsy table could now be integrated with the results of physical examination of the patient, and thus the diagnosis and prognosis of disease became more objective and precise.

Laënnec's fame as scientist, clinician and teacher spread over Europe and America. In 1822 he was appointed Regius Professor of Medicine at the Collège de France. Every weekday he conducted his rounds at the Hôpital de la Charité and taught for about two hours, much of the time in Latin, both because he thought this ought to be the universal language of science, and because many of his students were foreigners; his observations on patients were also written in Latin. But his health was failing rapidly. He suffered from dyspnea, cough, anorexia, weakness, faintings and great depression of spirits. This illness was called "nervous fever," but there is little doubt that he was then afflicted with phthisis. On several occasions he had recovered some strength by returning for more or less prolonged visits to his property of Kerlouarnec in Brittany and engaging there in the life of a country squire.

He was much impressed by the fact that phthisis was practically nonexistent among the peasants and small-town people around him, whereas it was the most important cause of death in Paris; he felt convinced that there was in the marine air something that protected from the disease. This conviction led him to advocate fresh air in the management of patients, and, contrary to the notions of the times, he insisted upon having the windows open day and night during his own illness. Imaginative and enterprising as ever, he had seaweed brought from

Brittany and spread on the floor around the beds of his wards in Paris. Infusions made of the weeds were given to the patients. For a time he had the illusion that these measures somewhat reduced cough and sputum, an example of the difficulties involved in evaluating methods of treatment of tuberculosis.

In May, 1825, Laënnec was attacked suddenly with fever, sweating, cough and a diarrhea. Auscultation with the stethoscope revealed pectoriloquy, the sign that phthisis had reached the dreaded cavity stage. Realizing that he could no longer stand the strain of his professional studies in Paris, he decided once more to retire to Brittany in the hope of a cure. The trip was exhausting and the patient was compelled to dose himself with opium to control diarrhea.

After ten days Kerlouarnec was reached, and Laënnec, craving the out-of-doors and a view of the farming country, rode in his carriage around the estate. The diarrhea and sputum waxed and waned; fever persisted. Despite weakness and the heat of July, Laënnec contrived to walk daily in the garden. During August, violent fever and delirium set in. On the last day of his life, during a moment of lucidity, he removed the rings from his fingers and placed them on a table, stating that he wanted to spare others this melancholy task. He then sank into a coma and expired a few hours later, in August, 1826.[4]

After Laënnec had shown that the tiny area of infiltration and the tubercle constitute the first phase of phthisis, the next question was to determine the origin of these primary alterations. Around 1850 the study of tissue cells in health and in disease began to dominate medical research. More and more emphasis was focused on the microscopic structure of the tubercle, which was found to consist of peculiar cells different from those present in normal tissues and in other disease states. As Lebert stated in 1843, "Whenever examinations with the naked eye leaves one in doubt as to the tuberculous, purulent or cancerous nature of a given lesion, the microscope will easily settle the issue."

Elaboration of this point of view occupied the attention of many eminent workers for several decades. In 1855 Rokitansky discovered the "giant cell," which he found to be one of the characteristic components of tubercles and which was further studied by Langhans in 1868. The most famous student of cellular pathology, Rudolph Virchow, contributed much to the knowledge of the cellular structure of tubercles, pointing out in particular the presence of lymphocytes and of the large epithelioid cells. Unfortunately, Virchow asserted also that only those lesions characterized by the typical gray, semitransparent tubercle were truly tuberculous, whereas those exhibiting caseation were of a different, nonspecific nature. In the same spirit, he stated that the caseating glandular lesions of scrofula were unrelated to true tuberculosis and merely the result of an inflammation due to some local "feebleness of the tissue." In other words, he claimed that tubercular phthisis differed in origin from caseous conditions, thus denying the unitarian theory expounded by Laënnec more than half a century before.

Virchow's views were wrong, but the very fact that he had been able to formulate and defend them points to a weakness in the edifice raised by Laënnec. The unitarian theory of phthisis was a brilliant concept based on precise observations of autopsy material; but Laënnec had never proved by experimentation that the different lesions of phthisis really did evolve one from the other in an orderly sequence, from the small tubercle, through the caseous ulcer, to the cavity stage. "How Laënnec hit on the facts," wrote one of his recent commentators, "we are unable to imagine. There is no doubt that he was either a superlative guesser or else an observer gifted in superlative degree with the power of generalization."

Laënnec could not prove his theory, because he did not know the primary cause of tuberculosis and, moreover, could not produce the disease at will in experimental animals. He was limited to the observation of its final results in the patient. The rigorous demonstration of Laënnec's inspired guess became possible only after techniques had been developed for the experimental production of the different forms of tuberculosis in laboratory animals.

CHAPTER VIII

The Germ Theory of Tuberculosis

THE BELIEF in the contagiousness of phthisis first became firmly entrenched, as we have seen, in Italy, Spain and the South of France. But the earliest explicit statement of the germ theory of disease before the microbiological era seems to have been formulated by a forgotten English physician, Benjamin Marten. In a volume printed in London in 1722 he presented his opinion that "animalculae fretting or gnawing the Vessels of the Stomach, Lungs, Liver" were the immediate cause of disease.

Having reviewed the factors believed by his contemporaries to be the cause of consumption, Marten suggested that these factors merely . . .

> . . . promote some other Peculiar, Latent or Essential Cause which I suppose to be joined with them. The Original and Essential Cause, then, which some content themselves to call a vicious Disposition of the Juices, others a Salt Acrimony, others a strange Ferment, others a Malignant Humour, may possibly be some certain Species of *Animalculae* or wonderfully minute living creatures that, by their peculiar Shape or disagreeable Parts are inimicable to our Nature; but, however, capable of subsisting in our Juices and Vessels.

One hundred and sixty years were to elapse before Koch actually saw the "minute living creatures" postulated by Marten, and proved them to be the cause of consumption. But today we are still much in the dark concerning the "peculiar shape" and "disagreeable parts" that make the tubercle bacilli so inimicable to our nature.

Marten reasonably deduced from his theory a number of conclusions which have stood the test of time. He suggested that . . .

> . . . the minute Animals or their Seed . . . are for the most part either conveyed from Parents to their Offspring hereditarily or communicated immediately from Distempered Persons to sound ones who are very conversant with them. . . . It may, therefore, be very likely that by habitual lying in the same Bed with a consumptive Patient, constantly eating and drinking with him or by very frequently conversing so nearly as to draw in part of the Breath he emits from the Lungs, a Consumption may be caught by a sound Person. . . . I imagine that slightly conversing with consumptive Patients is seldom or never sufficient to catch the Disease, there being but few if any of those minute Creatures . . . communicated in slender conversation.

This shrewd man knew well that a theory is of little use until documented and developed by facts and deeds. And wisely he presented his views as mere suggestions.

> I have said enough to evince the Reasonableness and Probability of my conjecture concerning the Prime and Essential Cause of Consumption as well as of many other Diseases; and to afford sufficient Hints to some abler hand whose abilities are more equal to the Task to carry the Theory much farther than I have done and, it may be, bring it to absolute Demonstration in an extensive Degree.

But the "hints" did not fall on fertile ground. Indeed, so unreceptive was eighteenth-century England to the contagion theory of phthisis that Marten's book was soon forgotten. When it was rediscovered in 1911, only four copies of it and very little concerning the life of the author could be found. It was not that the possibility of contagion was ignored by Marten's contemporaries, for throughout the eighteenth and early nineteenth century English and French physicians mention the theory in their writings, only to dismiss it as unsound. Many reasons account for their error. Microscopic organisms were known to occur in several parts of the body, but it was hard to understand at the time, and, indeed, it is still very unclear today, how "the fretting and gnawing" of these "animalculae" could bring about the tubercles, ulcers and huge cavities found in the phthisical patient. No form of reasoning could make the theory plausible *a priori.* And physicians can well be excused for having refused to believe in the germ causation of tuberculosis until compelled by the evidence of experimentation, by the gross fact that the disease, with its many types of lesions, could be produced at will by injecting a few bacteria into a normal animal.

The very prevalence of phthisis helped to obscure its contagious nature. It is certain that during the eighteenth and nineteenth centuries all dwellers in large cities of Europe became infected at an early age and remained in contact with heavily contaminated objects, sputum, food and dust throughout their life. However, infection does not necessarily mean disease, and phthisis became apparent chiefly in those afflicted with great natural susceptibility to it. Thus hereditary disposition overshadowed, and even completely masked, infectiousness.[1] On the other hand, the fact that the disease was rare in certain parts of the world while so prevalent in others, led physicians to conclude that it was the result of physiological disturbances caused by the environment. It was well known that tuberculous lesions in the lung often spread and invaded other organs, as if they had some infectious property; but this did not necessarily prove that they were caused by an infectious agent. It might merely mean that tuberculous tissue could graft itself onto healthy organs as does cancerous tissue. Indeed, Virchow regarded the tubercle as a tumor, and found no difficulty in accounting for its genesis, evolution, and structure in much the same terms that were used for the description of cancer.

Starting from the very same facts, it is easy now to arrive at conclusions opposite to those reached by Virchow and his school. If tuberculosis spreads from one organ to another, it is not because the tubercle grafts itself like a cancerous growth, but because the germs of tuberculosis are disseminated throughout the body by way of blood or lymph. If several brothers and sisters in a given family become tuberculous, it need not be the result of a special familial disposition, a phthisical diathesis, it may be simply that they have all been exposed to a heavy and continuous source of infection in the familial household. These explanations, however, are based on the germ theory of disease, and this theory did not become established in medical thinking until 1880.

It was the prevalence of tuberculosis among the Negroes in England that converted the English epidemiologist, William Budd, to the contagion theory of the disease. Negroes who contracted pulmonary phthisis while working on British ships were often sent to Clifton and Bristol for treatment. Budd wrote:

> The idea that phthisis . . . is disseminated through specific germs contained in the tuberculous matter cast off by persons already suffering from the disease first came into my mind . . . while I was walking on the Observatory Hill at Clifton in the second week of August 1856.
>
> Everywhere along the African sea-board, where the blacks have come into contact and intimate relations with the whites, phthisis causes a large mortality among them. In the interior, where intercourse with Europeans has been limited to casual contact . . . there is reason to believe that phthisis does not exist.

It was from the famous missionary, Dr. Livingstone, that Budd had learned that phthisis was practically unknown in the interior of Africa where the whites had not yet penetrated. Budd meditated eleven years before publishing his theory in the *Lancet* of October, 1867, and he does not seem to have contributed any specific information on the causation of tuberculosis.

During the same period, a French army surgeon, Jean-Antoine Villemin, took a fundamental step by demonstrating that phthisis is inoculable from man or cow to the rabbit and guinea pig, and can be transmitted from one infected animal to another in unending series. He presented this discovery for the first time before the French Academy of Medicine in 1865 and developed it in his great book, *Études sur la Tuberculose,* published in 1868. Villemin's experience as a military surgeon had made him aware of the fact that tuberculosis was more frequent among the medical personnel and soldiers stationed for long times in barracks than among troops in the field. He knew, furthermore, that healthy young men from country districts often became consumptive within a year or two after their arrival in army posts; and he also pointed out that prisoners, industrial workers and members of religious cloistered orders were more apt to contract the disease than were ordinary civilians.[2] All these observations reminded him of the fact that young and healthy horses would frequently die of the fulminating form of glanders when brought from isolated farms to depots where many horses were concentrated. The analogy was obvious to him and in simple, direct language he summarized his interpretation of the natural distribution of tuberculosis by the statement that "the phthisical soldier is to his messmates what the glandered horse is to its yoke fellow."

In fact, glanders in horses presents many similarities to tuberculosis in man, and knowing that the former disease could be transmitted by inoculation, Villemin resolved to prove that tuberculosis was also inoculable to animals. He introduced under the skin of young rabbits fragments of caseous material and fluid obtained from a man dead of phthisis. Three months later the animals were killed, and countless tubercles were found in their lungs and other organs. When rabbits were inoculated in a similar manner with tuberculous material obtained from a cow, a much more rapid and severe disease ensued. "It is remarkable," said Villemin, "that none of our rabbits, inoculated with human tuberculosis, has presented a disease so rapidly and completely generalized as that obtained by inoculation with the tubercle of the cow. . . . This would suggest that tuberculosis of bovine origin inoculated into the rabbit shows a greater activity than that of man inoculated into the same animal." Here was the first evidence that the germs of the human and bovine disease, otherwise so similar, differ in their virulence for the rabbit. As we shall see, the problem was to become the subject of a great international debate thirty years later when it was necessary to determine whether the germ of bovine tuberculosis could cause disease in man.

For several years Villemin accumulated evidence of the inoculability of tuberculosis to rabbits, guinea pigs, dogs, cats and other animals. He found that the sputum and sometimes the blood of patients contained the virulent principle. He proved also that the material taken from a scrofulous gland could induce in guinea pigs and rabbits the general picture of tuberculosis, thus demonstrating the etiological relation between scrofula and tuberculosis and giving to Laënnec's theory of the unity of phthisis the sanction of experimental evidence. Villemin's experiments demonstrated beyond doubt that tuberculosis does not originate spontaneously in man or animals as a result of emaciation, physiological misery, atmospheric disturbances, bad heredity, unhealthy occupations, or prolonged debilitating maladies. Its cause was some germ, living and multiplying in the body of the patient, and transmissible to a well person by direct contact or through the air.

Surprising as it may seem, Villemin's reports were received with such indifference that not even William Budd became aware of them. In part this was because the causation of disease by microorganisms had not yet been demonstrated. Even more, however, it was the belief in an innate susceptibility to tuberculosis which prevented the medical profession from being receptive to evidence of contagiousness.[3] The extent of this belief appears in the report of the commission appointed by the British Government to repeat Villemin's experiments. The English scientists inoculated fifty-three guinea pigs with tuberculous material and, in accordance with Villemin's claims, found that tubercles appeared in fifty of them. As controls they inserted setons of unbleached cotton in the shoulders of two other guinea pigs. One of these remained well, but the other died and was found riddled with lesions that appeared to be tuberculous. In the light of present knowledge, there is no question that the second animal either had been accidentally infected with tuberculosis by the inexperienced investigators, or had died from another disease, "pseudo-tuberculosis rodentium," which is common in guinea pigs. But this one exception was sufficient to rule out the theory of contagion in the minds of the investigators, and they worded accordingly the conclusions of their report, "M. Villemin's fact is established as unquestionable: certain of the lower animals, if inoculated from the human subject with the morbid products which are called 'tubercular,' will in consequence develop . . . a disease which is identical or nearly identical with the so-called 'tubercular' disease of man." But, the report went on, "A slight open wound such as that of a seton run beneath the skin . . . is capable of being the first step in a series of changes which gradually infect the creature's whole body with imitations of the human 'tubercular diathesis' and thus at last create such 'tubercular' disorganization as necessarily destroy life." Thus, the results in one guinea pig had been sufficient to bolster the official dogma of "diathesis" against the strength of all Villemin's inoculation experiments.[4]

Little by little, however, improved experimentation in Germany and in France added further evidence that tuberculosis was a specific, inoculable disease; and when the germ theory of disease gained widespread acceptance, the search for the germ of tuberculosis began in earnest. It seems certain that three German workers saw the tubercle bacillus in infected tissues almost simultaneously and independently in 1882. But so overwhelming was the mass of evidence, so masterly the experimentation, so convincing the demonstration presented by Robert Koch that to him goes the entire glory for demonstrating that tuberculosis is an infectious, bacillary disease.

In brief, Koch demonstrated the constant presence of the bacilli in the tuberculous lesions of men and animals; he cultivated these bacilli in pure culture on blood serum, and produced tuberculosis at will by inoculating the cultures into normal animals. These findings were first presented in a paper read before the Physiological Society of Berlin on March 24, 1882, then in a detailed description published in 1883, and later translated under the title, *The Etiology of Tuberculosis*. It seems that Villemin suffered much in his pride from seeing his work contemptuously ignored by Koch and all but forgotten by the rest of the world. He would have been wise to accept the cruel law of scientific life: "He becomes the true discoverer who establishes the truth: and the sign of the truth is the general acceptance. . . . In science the credit goes to the man who convinces the world, not to the man to whom the idea first occurs."

Koch was only thirty-nine when he discovered the tubercle bacillus.[5] While a medical officer in the small isolated town of Wollstein, he had started alone, with homemade equipment, his spectacular studies on contagious diseases. Anthrax of cattle was prevalent in the farms around him. In 1870 Koch startled the scientific world by reporting that he had found the bacteria that caused the disease, had cultivated them in the test tube, photographed them, followed their evolution throughout their life cycles, and produced anthrax by injecting them into laboratory animals. Then he had gained further laurels by developing techniques of elegant simplicity and perfection which are still in use today in bacteriological laboratories all over the world. In 1880, he was appointed Extraordinary Member of the Imperial Office of Health in Berlin, and director of a large laboratory staffed with devoted and skilled assistants. And now came the discovery of the causative agent of tuberculosis, a technical achievement of such magnitude that many consider it the greatest single feat of bacteriological science, one of the most important in the whole history of medicine.

Koch's work on tuberculosis produced such a phenomenal sensation among the lay public and in medical circles that it was immediately regarded as a landmark, indeed as heralding a new era in the study and control of the disease. Yet it did not propound a new conceptual scheme, for the germ theory of disease was already established. It did not offer a new approach to the problem of tuberculosis, for by 1882 the discovery of the microbial agent of the disease was considered only a question of time. The isolation of the tubercle bacillus did not require a new experimental methodology, for Koch merely had to modify details of techniques already worked out largely as the result of his own earlier work. Men were stunned by the practical import of the event, rather than by the intellectual effort involved in its genesis. What electrified the world was not the scientific splendor of the achievement, but rather the feeling that man had finally come to grips with the greatest killer of the human race. The "Captain of All the Men of Death" was no longer a vague phantom. The heretofore unseen killer was now visible as a living object, and its assailants at last had a target for their blows. In Europe and America Koch became the pope of medical science. In Japan a new shrine was dedicated to him, as to a demigod.[6]

The discovery and cultivation of the tubercle bacillus required the solution of technical problems which often baffle experienced bacteriologists even today. Koch started to search for the germ in gray tubercles that he crushed and stained by the classical techniques. Like others before him, he failed at first to see any microbial forms in the tubercles because the tubercle bacilli do not stain with dyes as readily as do other types of bacilli. Finally, successful results were obtained with an old preparation of methylene blue. Imaginative detective work led Koch to guess that the sample of dye that had proved effective had become contaminated with some of the ammonia present in the laboratory air, and this finding was the basis for the systematic use of alkali in the staining process. A slide preparation of infected tissue covered with dye was forgotten on the hot surface of a stove. Examination of the slide on the following day showed the bacilli brilliantly stained, and from then on heating became part of the routine staining technique. When a preparation that had been stained with methylene blue was counter-stained with Bismarck brown, everything on the slide became brown except the tubercle bacilli, which remained blue, and this differential staining characteristic was used to search for bacilli among tissue fragments.[7]

After many failures, the bacilli were grown on ox or sheep serum carefully sterilized and coagulated by heating at 65° C. But here again an unexpected finding presented itself. Whereas most other microbial species formed visible colonies in one or two days, tubercle bacilli grew much more slowly. Instead of discarding his preparations that appeared to remain sterile, Koch observed them day after day and finally was rewarded with the sight of minute colonies that became detectable with the hand lens after some ten days. These colonies proved to consist of bacilli that had the same morphological characteristics and peculiar staining properties as those seen in infected tissues of man or animals. Injection of pure cultures of these bacilli into guinea pigs by a great variety of methods produced typical tuberculosis. But Koch was not satisfied with a few tests to demonstrate the new fact. In his complete paper he presented records of bacteriological studies on ninety-eight cases of human and thirty-four cases of animal tuberculosis. He inoculated four hundred and ninety-six experimental animals, recovered forty-three pure bacillary cultures, and tested their virulence in two hundred animals.

Never had there been such a thorough piece of medical investigation.

In 1890, Koch released a new bombshell by announcing before the Tenth International Congress of Medicine in Berlin that he had discovered a substance that could protect against tuberculosis, and even cure the established disease. He refused at first to reveal the nature of the substance, which was referred to for a while as "Koch lymph," but under the pressure of public criticism he announced the following year that it was merely a glycerine extract of tubercle bacilli, the product now known under the name of "Old Tuberculin." [8] Koch's announcement of his discovery was heralded by headlines in all the leading medical publications. The English *Lancet* welcomed it in an editorial as "glad tidings of great joy," and the *British Medical Journal* was no less enthusiastic. Both journals published a complete translation of Koch's original article.

Excitement ran so high throughout the world that the publishers of the English *Review of Reviews* devoted almost the entire issue of December, 1890, to the event.[9]

> Europe [wrote the editor of the magazine] witnessed a strange but not unprecedented spectacle last month. In the Middle Ages the discovery of a new wonder-working shrine, or the establishment of the repute of the grave of a saint as a fount of miracles, often led to the same rush which has taken place last month to Berlin. . . . The consumptive patients of the Continent have been stampeding for dear life to the capital of Germany. The dying have hurried thither, sometimes to expire in the railway train, but buoyed up for a time by a new potent hope. . . .

Koch's announcement produced a profound sensation on the Mediterranean Riviera, that "last ditch of the consumptive."

> . . . The news that the German scientist had discovered a cure for consumption must have sounded as the news of the advent of Jesus of Nazareth in a Judaean village. The

whole community was moved to meet him. His fame went throughout the region around about, and telegrams in the newspapers announced that all the sleeping cars had been engaged for months to come to convey the consumptives of the Riviera to the inclement latitude of Berlin.

The first English physician to arrive in Berlin after the announcement of Koch's discovery was A. Conan Doyle.[10] Even then a famous writer, he was still practicing medicine. The details of his visit to Berlin, published in the *Review of Reviews*, are of interest in depicting the atmosphere of worship surrounding the personality of the illustrious German scientist who, like the "veiled Prophet . . . remains unseen to any eyes save those of his own immediate co-workers." To Conan Doyle, Koch appeared as . . .

> . . . a man so devoted to his own particular line of work, that all descriptions of him from other points of view must, in the main, be negative. Some five feet and a half in height, sturdily built, with brown hair fringing off to grey at the edges, he is a man whose appearance might be commonplace were it not for the vivacity of his expression and the quick decision of his manner.

In the same article, Conan Doyle presents a statement of the mode of action, potential usefulness, limitations and dangers of tuberculin of such intelligent understanding that little of importance has since been added to his analysis of the subject.

> Koch has never claimed that his fluid kills the tubercle bacillus. On the contrary, it has no effect upon it, but destroys the low form of tissue in the meshes of which the bacilli lie. Should this tissue slough in the case of lupus, or be expelled in the sputum in the case of phthisis, and should it contain in its meshes all the bacilli, then it would be possible to hope for a complete cure. When one considers, however, the number and the minute size of these deadly organisms, and the evidence that the lymphatics as well as the organs are affected by them, it is evident that

> it will only be in very exceptional cases that the bacilli are all expelled. Your remedy does not treat the real seat of the evil. It continually removes the traces of the enemy, but it still leaves him deep in the invaded country.

Moreover, Doyle pointed out, it often happens that treatment with tuberculin . . .

> . . . stirs into activity all those tubercular centres which have become dormant. In one case which I have seen, the injection, given for the cure of a tubercular joint, caused an ulcer of the eye, which had been healed for twenty years, to suddenly break out again, thus demonstrating that the original ulcer came from a tubercular cause. It may also be remarked that the fever after the injection is in some cases so very high (41° C.) . . . that it is hardly safe to use it in the case of a debilitated patient.

Doyle concluded his analysis by expressing much doubt as to the usefulness of tuberculin in therapy, but he prognosticated that the substance would prove of great use in diagnosis.

> Tubercle, and tubercle alone, responds to its action, so that in all cases where the exact nature of a complaint is doubtful, a single injection is enough to determine whether it is scrofulous, lupous, phthisical, or in any way tuberculous. This alone is a very important addition to the art of medicine.

Doyle's anticipations were amply confirmed by subsequent events. It soon became obvious that tuberculin killed many more patients than it helped, and the treatment fell in discredit almost everywhere. In 1884, one year after the glowing account of the discovery of tuberculin, the *British Medical Journal* published a scathing article condemning Koch for his unethical behavior in having attempted to keep secret the composition of the substance, and for his lack of scientific judgment in having recommended it as a remedy. Nevertheless Koch's work had not been in vain, for, as Doyle had foreseen, tuberculin was to prove before long a most useful tool in the detection of tuberculous infection.[11]

In his paper announcing the ill-starred "cure," Koch also presented a careful description of some experiments that have become the basis of much later work on the immunological aspects of tuberculosis. Instead of reporting these experiments in detail, it seems best to analyze how their results contributed to the understanding and control of tuberculosis.

When virulent tubercle bacilli are injected into the skin of a normal guinea pig, they produce at first only little reaction, and the scar heals after a few days. The bacilli, however, immediately start to multiply and invade the various organs of the body. Some two to three weeks later, there appears at the site of injection a nodule which ulcerates, and the ulcer remains open until the animal's death. A very different response is observed if a second dose of living bacilli is injected into the skin of the same guinea pig several weeks after the initial infection. The site of the second injection becomes inflamed within one to two days, but the newly formed ulcer heals quickly. Moreover, many of the bacilli of the second dose appear to be destroyed at the site of injection, while those of the original infection continue to multiply in other parts of the body and eventually kill the animal. This obscure and complex set of events is known under the name of "Koch phenomenon." It illustrates the puzzling fact, still poorly understood, that the tuberculous individual offers much resistance to a new infection, although often unable to overcome the original disease. We shall see later how these facts have led to the development of a technique of preventive vaccination against tuberculosis.

In the same paper Koch reported that the difference in reactivity between the normal and the tuberculous individual can also be made evident by injecting into them bacilli killed by heat or chemicals, or extracts of bacilli such as the soluble preparation which he called tuberculin. Tuberculin produces little, if any, reaction when injected into a normal animal or man. But it behaves as a powerful poison and may even cause death if injected in sufficient quantities in a tuberculous individual. It is that fact, as already noted, which renders it so dangerous for the treatment of tuberculosis. Only tubercle bacilli (or certain of their products) are capable of "sensitizing" the body to the toxic effect of tuberculin. Thus, tuberculosis brings about in the diseased person a change which expresses itself by an increased and specific reactivity to the products of tubercle bacilli. According to present-day parlance, the tuberculous body is *allergic* to these products.

Much is now known of tuberculin allergy. Of particular importance is the fact that it appears long before any other obvious sign of disease, and that it persists for years after the active phase of the disease has ended. Even when the tuberculous infection remains so mild as to be almost symptomless, allergy develops just the same and may last for years. Thus, the finding that an individual gives a positive tuberculin test is convincing evidence that he is or has been infected, but does not necessarily indicate that he is suffering from active disease. As will be shown later these facts are of great help in studying the prevalence of tuberculosis and in controlling its spread.

The tuberculin sensitivity test is carried out by applying tuberculin (or a purified derivative of it known as PPD) under, in or on the skin. Because the test material may elicit severe reactions in the allergic individual, it is injected in exceedingly small amounts, usually in several graded doses. Koch himself experienced these toxic reactions following the injection into his arm of a fairly heavy dose of tuberculin. He described his symptoms in the following words: "Drawing pains in the extremities, lassitude, tendency to cough, difficulty in breathing which rapidly increased, during the fifth hour an unusually violent chill which lasted almost one hour accompanied by nausea, vomiting, fever up to 39° C." Fortunately, these dramatic symptoms progressively subsided, and the hero of the celebrated experiment was back to normal after a few days. Koch was a vigorous, healthy man, and there is no evidence that he ever suffered from tuberculosis. But the account of his response to the injection of tuberculin leaves no doubt that he, too, had been infected, at some time – having probably regarded as malaise, mere cold, or grippe an undiagnosed bout with tubercle bacilli in his youth.

Following Villemin's original observations, there had been many reports pointing to some difference between the types of germs causing tuberculosis in man and in cattle. Careful studies differentiating the two types had been presented by the American bacteriologist, Theobald Smith. In 1901, in a lecture delivered before the British Congress on Tuberculosis, Koch reported experiments showing that human tubercle bacilli do not produce progressive disease in cattle. Whether bovine bacilli are as innocuous for man as human bacilli are for cattle was more difficult to determine since experimentation with human beings was out of the question. Koch pointed out, however, that man ingested large numbers of bacilli of the bovine type present in the milk, cream and butter from tuberculous cows. Believing that the bovine type of tuberculosis is very rare in man he reached the tentative conclusion that man is probably as resistant to bovine tuberculosis as cattle are resistant to human tuberculosis.

This was merely an opinion based on circumstantial evidence, but an opinion expressed by Koch carried the authority of law in many quarters. The statement was of enormous practical importance since it seemed to justify the use of tuberculous milk for human consumption, and immediately those who believed in the virulence of bovine bacilli for man took issue with Koch. In fact, a thorough examination of the problem, undertaken by several groups of workers, in particular by the English Royal Commission on Tuberculosis, soon established beyond doubt that, contrary to Koch's belief, tuberculosis of bovine type was a serious problem in man and particularly in children. The campaigns for the pasteurization of milk and for the eradication of bovine tuberculosis were the practical outcomes of this discovery.

In addition to tubercle bacilli of the human and bovine type, a few others have been recognized. Bacilli of the avian type are highly pathogenic for birds, hogs, and rabbits, but rarely found in man or cattle. Bacilli of the murine type are the cause of a widespread infection of field mice (voles) in England. Bacilli of the piscine type produce tuberculous lesions in cold-blooded animals such as frogs. Furthermore, there exist in nature a large variety of microorganisms which are members of the so-called acid-fast family like the true tubercle bacilli, but are never found in disease conditions; they occur in the mud of ditches, in oil deposits, on rubber tubings, in butter, on hay, and often in large numbers on certain parts of the body.

The differentiation of these various microbial types has completed the phase of the germ theory of tuberculosis concerned with identifying the causative agents of the disease. Analysis of the mechanisms by which true tubercle bacilli bring about the lesions, signs, and symptoms of tuberculosis is the focus of attention during the present phase. To deal with this problem bacteriologists have undertaken chemical and physiological investigations of components, products and activities of the bacilli in the hope of discovering the primary cause of the abnormal reactions which they elicit. From these studies will certainly emerge a broader interpretation of the germ theory of disease. Going deeper than the anatomical lesion, and beyond the tubercle bacillus, it will reach the subtle biochemical reactions by which the microorganisms cause specific functional disturbances in the cells and tissues of the infected individual.

CHAPTER IX

Infection and Disease

TUBERCLE BACILLI are minute rods, so small that large numbers of them can be packed inside the microscopic white cells of the blood and tissues. In fact, they are readily engulfed by these white cells, in health as well as in disease. When cultivated in the test tube, they multiply at a very slow rate even in the most favorable nutrient broths. They produce a new generation approximately twice a day, some twenty times slower than most other microorganisms, and it appears that their rate of multiplication is also relatively slow in the tissues and body fluids during infection. They have little ability to break down complex organic molecules and are incapable of attacking many of the substances that form the structural components of our organs. Yet, despite all these biochemical limitations, they reach enormous numbers in the tissues that they invade, and their presence in the body results in the huge ulcers and cavities that give to tuberculosis its peculiar and dramatic character.

What properties do tubercle bacilli possess that permit them to establish themselves, multiply, and do damage in the human body? In other words, what is the mechanism of tuberculous disease?

Benjamin Marten was not far from the truth when he suggested that his hypothetical "animalculae" caused disease by virtue of the fact that their "disagreeable Parts are inimicable to our Nature." Modern research is attempting to restate his hypothesis in the words of pathology and biochemistry. It is known that infection with living tubercle bacilli is not the only method for producing the lesions of tuberculosis; the same result can be obtained by injecting into experimental animals dead bacilli, or fragments or soluble extracts of them. In other words, the lesions of tuberculosis are brought about, not because the bacilli possess the property of life, but because their constituents and products exert a toxic, irritating effect on our tissues, because indeed "their Parts are inimicable to our Nature." Thus, certain fractions of the dead bacilli elicit the production of characteristic tubercles, whereas others render the animals allergic to tuberculin; injection of large amounts of bacillary material can cause the appearance of ulcers full of caseous material, and even bring about a state of chronic toxemia, with progressive emaciation resulting in death. Progress is slowly being made towards the chemical identification of the bacillary constituents responsible for all these dramatic effects. It has even been possible to produce tuberculous-like lesions by injecting, into animals, substances synthesized in the chemical laboratory in imitation of those found in the bacilli. One may well expect that a time will come when the manifestations of tuberculosis can be traced to the toxic effects exerted on body structures and functions by bacillary substances of known chemical nature.

Although it is possible to elicit detectable lesions with dead bacilli or their products, this can be done only by injecting large quantities of material — the amounts must be many million times larger than the mass of living bacilli present in an infective dose sufficient to cause disease under natural conditions. The small numbers of bacilli present in a droplet of infected sputum, or in the milk from a tuberculous cow, cannot by themselves produce extensive lesions; they only initiate the infectious process. To be able to elicit the signs and symptoms of tuberculosis, they must multiply enormously in the tissues of the person who has inhaled the sputum or consumed the milk. In other words, disease under natural conditions occurs only if the bacilli undergo multiplication after they have been introduced into the body and if they manufacture sufficient amounts of the irritating and toxic materials which are directly responsible for the symptoms and lesions.

Fortunately, most of the bacilli with which we come in contact are not capable of multiplying extensively in our tissues. Even though they can survive there for prolonged periods of time, they cannot initiate the disease process. In other words, they are not virulent for man. It would be, needless to say, of much theoretical interest and probably of the greatest practical importance to know what peculiarities in structure and properties are responsible for the virulence of certain types of bacilli, but this is still shrouded in mystery.

It is obvious that, in order to multiply, the bacilli must first be able to survive the onslaught of all the destructive agents to which they are subjected in the body. In general, microorganisms reaching the tissues soon encounter a series of defense mechanisms which tend to eliminate or destroy them. It is axiomatic, therefore, that virulent tubercle bacilli possess some structures or attributes capable of protecting them. As they are known to produce peculiar fatty substances which cover their surfaces, it has been postulated, but without adequate proof, that these materials shield them from certain antimicrobial effects of the tissue cells and humors. Be that as it may, survival is not enough. The bacilli must increase in numbers.

Ability to multiply requires a very fine adjustment between the growth requirements of the bacilli and the conditions prevailing in the tissues. A striking illustration of this statement was brought to light recently by a group of Australian investigators. While studying cases of severely destructive skin ulcers occurring in man, they found in the lesions large numbers of bacilli which at first could not be differentiated from true tubercle bacilli. For a long time, however, all attempts to grow the skin bacilli in the test tube gave negative results – until one day cultures were obtained through a happy accident: the thermostatic control of the incubator had failed to function, and the temperature had fallen to 34° C. instead of being maintained at 37.5° C., which is that of the inner parts of the body. Systematic investigation revealed the unexpected fact that the ulcer bacilli could multiply only at a few degrees below 37.5° C. When injected into the veins of experimental animals, they produce lesions only on the body surfaces where the temperature is lowered by contact with the outside atmosphere, but not in the inner organs. Here then is a case where limitation of virulence seems to be due to peculiar temperature requirements.

There are many other unidentified factors, more subtle and probably more important, that play a part in determining virulence, but our ignorance of the subject is so complete that it is best to acknowledge it instead of presenting hypotheses that have little basis in fact. Nor do we have any clearer picture of the process by which the body attempts to interfere with multiplication of the virulent bacilli, or to overcome their toxic effects.

And yet, it is certain that there come into play in the course of infection powerful defense mechanisms, which often succeed in bringing about arrest of the disease, complete or partial, temporary or permanent.

When virulent bacilli reach the tissues of a susceptible individual who has never been tuberculous before, they start multiplying at once and continue to increase in numbers for at least several weeks. In most human beings the infection then comes to a standstill, even though living, virulent bacilli survive in the tissues for many years. Obviously, the infection has brought about a certain state of resistance that checks its further progress, but this resistance is not absolute, and its duration is uncertain. In many cases, introduction of new bacilli from the outside several years later will initiate a new focus of disease in an individual who had once been able to arrest a well-established lesion. Furthermore, a lesion which has long remained dormant, but still contains living bacilli, may become active again, as if some restraining influences which had held the bacilli in check became ineffective with time.

Control of the disease process can probably be brought about by several different mechanisms, either by interfering with the multiplication of the bacilli, or by neutralizing their ability to cause damage to the infected tissues. It is certain that the factors which determine susceptibility or resistance to tuberculosis are controlled by heredity, become modified by living conditions, and probably have as their basis some of the processes of immunity which operate in other infectious diseases. But, surprising as it may seem, no technique is presently available to identify, or measure, any of the hereditary or acquired characteristics which determine the course of tuberculosis in human beings or even in experimental animals. In contrast with this lack of understanding of the controlling factors of susceptibility to tuberculosis, there exists a large body of descriptive knowledge concerning the different phases of the infection.

In general, bacilli first reach the air sacs of the lungs after being inhaled in droplets of sputum or in particles of dust. More rarely, the intestines are the first seat of infection, as a result of ingestion of contaminated food. From these initial foci, the bacilli are transported by way of the blood stream to the different parts of the body. There is reason to believe that in a small percentage of cases the infection spreads rapidly, causing an acute, fatal disease with signs and symptoms so unspecific that proper diagnosis is not made. In other cases it manifests itself in the more obvious form of miliary tuberculosis. More commonly, however, the disease follows a chronic, protracted course.

Following primary infection, the bacilli are immediately engulfed by the white cells of the blood and of the tissues and multiply probably within them. They seem to cause little if any damage at first and do not call forth any remarkable reaction. From the site of penetration they are soon transported by way of the lymph channels to the nearest lymph node and multiply there also, but still the infection produces no striking symptoms. Within several weeks or a very few months, however, the continued presence of the bacilli in ever-increasing numbers brings about the remarkable alteration already described under the name of tuberculin allergy. Many of the tissue cells that have become hypersensitive to the bacilli and their products are killed by mere contact with them.[1]

Once allergy has become established, a number of dramatic changes take place in the areas invaded by the bacilli. The inflammation is intense, and it manifests itself by an outpouring of cells and fluid from the blood vessels located around the infected site. On the other hand, a new type of tissue begins to organize itself around the bacilli, as if to wall them off. The cluster of tissue cells surrounding the infected area constitutes the microscopic tubercle which continues to expand for a while by pushing aside the normal tissue, or by coalescing with adjacent tubercles. The further evolution of the tubercle is extremely complex, and is determined by the relative activities of several independent processes. A network of fibrous tissue may form around it and isolate it more or less completely from the rest of the body. The allergic cells which are killed by the bacilli or their products break up into a mass of cheeselike debris. In certain cases this caseous material softens and takes the appearance of pus. In others, the tubercle eventually becomes impregnated with fibrous tissue and later with calcium, thus being transformed into a hard nodule. In reality, all these processes may occur in the same person either at different times or often simultaneously in different parts of the body, thus giving rise to the confused picture which so much perplexed the anatomopathologists of past centuries and which is still almost as much of a puzzle today.

The characteristic lesion, consisting of the patch of lung tissue first affected and of the infected caseous lymph node associated with it, is usually designated the primary complex. Although this stage of the disease is accompanied by much tissue damage, the patient often is unaware of any symptoms, or these are so slight that they are dismissed as a cold or grippe. The amount of lung tissue destroyed is too small to affect pulmonary ventilation in a significant manner.

The subsequent evolution of the disease is extremely complicated and unpredictable. Under the most favorable circumstances, the lesion does not spread further; it may become encapsulated and eventually calcified. Even then, however, living, virulent bacilli persist in the tuberculous tissue for prolonged periods of time, constituting for years a potential source of reactivation of disease.

If the lesion remains caseous and active, it will eventually soften by penetration into it of the liquid and cellular elements of the blood. When the lesion breaks open into a bronchus, the discharge of its softened contents into these channels leaves a hole, a cavity, in the lung tissue. The secondary consequences of this event are far more dangerous than cavitation itself. For the living bacilli and the toxic materials that are forced out from the lesion into the blood vessels or bronchi become disseminated in other parts of the body and start new foci of tuberculosis.

Dissemination by way of the blood may give rise to forms of the disease with a rapidly fatal course, miliary tuberculosis or tuberculous meningitis for example, as well as to destructive lesions of the kidneys and of the bones. Erosion into the bronchi results in spread of the infection to new areas of the lung and often also to the larynx and the intestines. The new foci of infection need not evolve into fatal disease and may in their turn stop spreading and become encapsulated. As the amount of lung tissue possessed by the normal individual is far in excess of that required for ordinary physical activities, tuberculosis is not incompatible with a normal span of life if it remains localized in the lung. Nevertheless, each relapse results in the destruction of more lung tissue, and interferes further with pulmonary ventilation, besides increasing the danger of generalized and fatal spread of the disease.

The biographical sketches of consumptive individuals given in earlier chapters illustrate the fact that, until the first decades of the twentieth century, tuberculosis was diagnosed only after it had reached an advanced stage. Coughing, spitting of blood, hectic fever, night sweats, emaciation and pallor are always the manifestations of extensive damage and of the toxic reactions produced in the allergic individual by the adsorption of bacillary components and of breakdown products from dead tissues.

In his *Essay on the Causes, Early Signs of, and Prevention of Pulmonary Consumption,* published in 1799, Thomas Beddoes presents a clinical picture of the consumptive patient which was at that time regarded as characteristic of the disease:

> The emaciated figure strikes one with terror; the forehead covered with drops of sweat; the cheeks painted with a livid crimson, the eyes sunk; the little fat that raised them in their orbits entirely wasted; the pulse quick and tremulous; the nails long, bending over the ends of the fingers; the palms of the hand dry and painfully hot to the touch; the breath offensive, quick and laborious, and the cough so incessant as scarce to allow the wretched sufferer time to tell his complaints.

It is probable that there had long been some awareness of the fact that patients display these symptoms only in the advanced stages of consumption. Oddly enough, Niccolò Machiavelli alluded to it in the fifteenth century in an unexpected comparison between the management of affairs of state and the treatment of tuberculosis:

> . . . Consumption . . . in the commencement is easy to cure, and difficult to understand; but when it has neither been discovered in due time, nor treated upon a proper principle, it becomes easy to understand, and difficult to cure. The same thing happens in state affairs, by foreseeing them at a distance, which is only done by men of talents, the evils which might arise from them are soon cured; but when, from want of foresight, they are suffered to increase to such a height that they are perceptible to everyone, there is no longer any remedy.

It is only during recent decades, however, that the importance of detecting the disease during its very early phase has been generally recognized; and the development of more effective diagnostic techniques constitutes probably the most important contribution of medical science to the control of tuberculosis.

To place the problem in its proper light it seems worth considering for a moment the significance of the term "disease." Etymologically speaking, the meaning seems simple and clear enough; the *dis-eased* person is one who is not at ease because of disturbing symptoms. And this definition provides the key to one of the most dangerous aspects of tuberculosis. The symptoms during the early phase being vague, they are usually dismissed as trivial malaise unrelated to pulmonary lesions, and the tuberculous process can become very extensive before the patient really feels *diseased.*[2] It is the realization of this fact which has stimulated the search for diagnostic methods not dependent upon subjective symptoms.

All through the nineteenth century clinicians continued to develop the techniques of percussion and auscultation and learned to derive from them even more diagnostic clues than had been thought possible by Auenbrugger and Laënnec. The techniques of physical diagnosis reached an extreme degree of refinement and accuracy, or illusion of accuracy. The masters of the art compared the various chest sounds to the sound of silk or wool, new or old leather, or other esoteric objects, and they related each of them to a particular disease process. Eventually, however, a reaction took place against these exaggerated claims of diagnostic acumen, and Osler took a malicious pleasure in quoting the physician who had written him in all seriousness, "I am sending you a patient who has a cavity at the top of the right lung the size of a walnut *without the shell.*" But, on the whole, percussion and auscultation long remained the essential techniques of the diagnostician. Some progress came with the use of the laryngoscope and bronchoscope, which permitted visualization of the larynx and bronchi.[3] By far the most important advance, however, was the use of X rays, which rendered possible the detection of abnormal densities in many organs and particularly in the lungs, kidneys, nodes and gastro-intestinal tract.

It is entertaining to muse over the circumstances under which the penetrating power of X rays was discovered. One might imagine committees appointed to organize large research laboratories with all kinds of specialized scientists and to formulate logical research programs, with the purpose of developing techniques for the visualization of the inner parts of the human body. Instead, Roentgen discovered X rays in 1895 as an accidental by-product of experiments designed for an entirely different purpose. He was studying the phenomena of electric discharge in the high vacuum of a Crookes tube when he noticed a black line being produced on a piece of barium-platino-cyanide paper separated from the tube by a shield of black cardboard. He had the curiosity to trace the origin of this effect and recognized by a few experiments that it was produced by rays capable of penetrating the cardboard. These were the X rays.

The discovery immediately produced a tremendous sensation

throughout the world, a firm in London exploiting it as early as 1896 to the extent of advertising "X-ray-proof" underwear! For a time the utilization of the penetrating power of the rays for diagnosis was treated with scorn by conservative physicians, just as had been percussion, and auscultation with the stethoscope. But the potential usefulness of the discovery soon became obvious, and it was not long before fluoroscopy, then stereoscopic X-ray examination of the chest, became accepted as powerful procedures for the diagnosis of disease.

Roentgenograms (X-ray photographs) permit the detection of tuberculous lesions long before the patient is aware of any subjective symptoms. They also make it possible to gain some idea of the character, extent and age of these lesions, and to follow their course. But, despite its immense help in the diagnosis of tuberculosis, roentgenology leaves many questions unanswered. It does not yet allow detection of the very early lesions, and, conversely, lesions that appear to be healed according to the X-ray picture often retain active soft parts containing living bacilli. Thus, the method is not sensitive and accurate enough to give to the physician some of the most necessary information.

It is well recognized, furthermore, that the abnormalities revealed by X rays can be caused by diseases other than tuberculosis, such as fungus infections or cancer. Final diagnosis must rest, therefore, on more specific techniques. The most convincing of all is the demonstration of tubercle bacilli by bacteriological methods. This is fairly easy when the bacilli are sufficiently numerous to be seen by direct microscopic examination of sputum or other pathological specimens. When bacilli are too few for visual detection, resort must be had, for the demonstration of their presence, to cultivation of the suspected material on artificial culture media or to its injection into guinea pigs. Unfortunately, these methods are time-consuming and not always reliable. It seems probable that immunological procedures utilizing blood or skin tests could give useful information, as they have in other infectious diseases; but they are still in their infancy. The development of efficient procedures for early diagnosis remains today one of the practical problems of tuberculosis most in need of imaginative study.

Imperfect as they are, modern diagnostic techniques have brought out the fundamental facts that many human beings are infected with tubercle bacilli without being aware of it and that the infection often subsides spontaneously without causing any obvious trouble. This situation had been anticipated by Richard Morton. After observing the frequent occurrence of tubercles in cadavers, he wrote in his *Phthisiologia:*

> Yea, when I consider with myself, how often in one year there is cause enough ministered for producing these swellings, even to those who are wont to observe the strictest mode of living, I cannot sufficiently admire that any one, at least after he comes to the flower of his youth, can die without a touch of consumption.
>
> And without doubt the breeding of these swellings is so frequent and common, that a consumption of the lungs would necessarily be the common plague of mankind, if these swellings did not vanish . . . as easily as they are bred at first.

Surveys made at the beginning of the twentieth century revealed that almost all members of the adult population in European and American cities were tuberculin positive and, therefore, had been at some time infected with tubercle bacilli. Examination with X rays added to the significance of this finding by showing evidence of active tuberculous lesions in many individuals who were thought to be normal and healthy.

In 1926 there occurred in Lübeck, Germany, a tragedy that constituted an experimental demonstration of the phenomenal resistance exhibited by most human beings to tuberculous infection. Through a mistake, two hundred and forty-nine babies who were to be vaccinated were given instead enormous numbers of living, virulent tubercle bacilli of the human type. Of these babies, seventy-six died of acute tuberculous disease, but one hundred and seventy-three developed only minor lesions and survived the infection. When last observed twelve years later, the survivors were still free of tuberculosis.

The physical basis of susceptibility and resistance is a much debated question. It is often claimed that certain human stocks — for example, those with blue eyes and red hair, or most of the colored races — are particularly susceptible to tuberculosis; but this relation has not been convincingly substantiated. As we shall see later, differences in susceptibility between different ethnic groups do exist, but they depend upon the extent to which the group has lived in contact with tubercle bacilli in the past, rather than upon racial origin.

On the basis of practical experience, the early physicians had come to the view that certain physical types of human beings are more prone than others to suffer from tuberculosis. The first classical description of the *typus phthisicus* dates from Hippocrates, and many subsequent authors have given slightly modified versions of it. Wrote Christopher Bennet, in the seventeenth century:

> Nor are there wanting such as bring their consumption with them into the World, whose Parents have died Valetudinarians or Consumptive. . . . These Persons have sharp shoulders which are therefore called wing-like, a contracted Thorax, a narrow and low Chest, a thin, long neck, a flaccid Tone of all the Parts about the Breast and a very flabby Contexture of the muscles all over the Body.

It is now realized that destructive processes in the lungs bring about changes in the shape of the chest. Since, until recently, the prolonged, smoldering forms of the disease remained undiagnosed as long as they did not cause dramatic symptoms, many patients developed the anatomical abnormalities of *habitus phthisicus* before they became obviously ill. In reality, therefore, the *habitus phthisicus* can be of little help in indicating those likely to develop the disease – since it is often the result rather than the inciting cause of tuberculosis.

Much has been written, also, throughout the ages, of an alleged relation of the tuberculous type to "genius, passion and delicate sensibility." But here again, the evidence is far from convincing. Long ago, Benjamin Marten expressed the skeptical attitude in his usual felicitous manner:

> The divine Hippocrates and from him several others tell us that Persons with a fine Contexture, tender, and who have a small shrill Voice, thin clear Skin, a long Neck, narrow Breast, depressed or strait Chest and whose shoulder blades stick out are of all others most subject to Consumption; and this is in some measure confirmed by Experience but must not be taken as a general Rule because we often find robust and strong men fall into this Distemper and such weakly tender Persons as above described many times exempted from it.
>
> Consumptive People are likewise generally observed to be very full of Spirit, hasty and of a sharp and ready Wit. . . . But that only ingenious Men are seized with this Distemper cannot be said.

The unquestionable and all-important fact remains, however, that infection does not necessarily mean progressive disease and that individuals differ greatly in their ability to overcome it. The often observed prevalence of tuberculosis in certain families suggests that hereditary factors affect natural susceptibility and resistance. This appears particularly evident in the study of tuberculosis in identical twins. It has been found that if one twin becomes tuberculous, the other also is likely to develop tuberculosis and to exhibit a type of disease with a similar course. This similarity of disease is frequently observed even if the identical twins are separated early in life and exposed to infection under very different circumstances. Still more convincing, and probably more useful for the future development of knowledge, is the experimental breeding of families of rabbits and guinea pigs exhibiting a predictable and uniform resistance to infection. It is much to be hoped that the comparative study of these breeds of animals will give clues for the recognition and measurement of the factors that control the outcome of tuberculous infection in human beings.

There are many facts substantiating the view that general physiological factors have a profound, indeed a dominant, effect on resistance to tuberculosis, whatever the degree of exposure to infection. The relation of mortality to age is a case in point, for it has long been recognized that the mortality from tuberculosis is much lower in children of the age group from five to puberty than in younger or older individuals. The phenomenon is so striking that the favored years have come to be referred to as "the golden age" of resistance to tuberculosis.

The low mortality in the five-to-fifteen age group was already obvious in 1900, at a time when immense numbers of babies and young adults were dying of tuberculosis and when infection was well-nigh universal. Today, the relation between age and disease can still be readily recognized among the colored people in the United States; children of school age only rarely exhibit signs of progressive and fatal disease despite intimate associations with adults afflicted by it. It is certain, therefore, that greater resistance and not lack of contact with bacilli accounts for the lower death rates of the young adolescents. This greater resistance may exist partly because society provides for young people an environment where they are protected to some extent against many of the stresses and ordeals of life. But it is likely, also, that during the years before puberty the physiological and hormonal make-up can mobilize forces that retard the progress of tuberculous disease. Worth pointing out in this respect is the fact that the years from five to fifteen are the "golden age" not only with reference to tuberculosis, but to other infections as well. For instance, young adolescents are also resistant to bronchitis and pneumonia, and to the ill-defined conditions entered under the name of diarrhea and enteritis on death certificates.[4] (Appendices D and E.)

A study carried out over a period of some twenty-five years at the Children's Chest Clinic of Bellevue Hospital in New York has provided very important information concerning the fate of individuals who *contract* tuberculosis during childhood. More than 23 per cent of the young patients coming from poor, overcrowded homes died within a few months, as a direct result of primary infection. Of infants first diagnosed when six months of age, 55 per cent died as against 28 per cent of the infants one to two years old, and only 15 per cent of the group four to nine years old. Within fourteen years after they had apparently recovered from their primary infection, 8 per cent of the survivors developed pulmonary tuberculosis. Of particular interest is the fact that this late complication occurred twice as frequently among girls as among boys. In the majority of girls, pulmonary lesions were first found in the age group of thirteen to fifteen years, with a striking relation to the onset of menses.

Thus, many independent lines of evidence suggest that resistance to tuberculosis is affected in some obscure manner by physiological factors associated with growth and adolescence. But even though it appears that children of five to fifteen years old are less likely to die of tuberculosis than younger or older individuals, nevertheless it is also true that infection contracted in that age period entails great dangers for the future. The evidence seems inescapable that in many cases the fatal phthisis of early or late adulthood is the delayed phase of an infection contracted during the "golden age," which manifested itself at first as a trivial malaise.

In addition to the innate physiological characteristics determined by heredity and age, there are many environmental influences which modify the manner in which the body responds to infection. The effects of fatigue, nutrition, housing and climate will be considered later. Psychic reactions also must be given an important place among the conditioning factors of disease.[5] "It is just as important to know what is in a man's head as what is in his chest," said Osler, "if you want to predict the outcome of his pulmonary tuberculosis."

This statement echoes an opinion expressed countless times in every period and every land by physicians interested in the causation of tuberculosis. Wrote Morton, "I have very often observed that a consumption of the lungs has had its origin from long and grievous passions of the mind." In a similar vein, C. G. Hufeland asserted in 1797 that a "mournful disposition of the soul" was one of the causes of scrofula. A few years later, Auenbrugger put the blame on "affections of the mind, particularly ungratified desires, the principal of which is nostalgia," and Laënnec wrote of "profound, melancholy passions, extending over long periods of time."[6]

The modern physician shies away from these vague assertions. Instead, he describes case after case in which some severe psychic disturbance, such as caused by an unhappy love affair, a familial tragedy, or financial difficulties, is followed a few weeks or a few months later by an attack or a recurrence of tuberculosis. If he is so trained, he will use the vocabulary of psychosomatic medicine to explain the striking correlation between what goes on in the head and what goes on in the chest. When understanding fails, one is reduced to inventing new words.[7] For in reality, little if anything has been added to what had already been perceived by the physicians of past centuries. In tuberculosis, as in other fields of medicine, it remains for the future to unravel the subtle mechanisms by which the psyche and the soma influence each other.[8]

The word "tuberculosis," it will be recalled, was introduced during the first half of the nineteenth century to denote a group of diseases characterized by the production of tubercles in different parts of the body. After the discovery that tuberculous lesions were caused by a particular type of microorganism, the meaning of the word underwent an evolution that expressed the shift from the purely anatomical to the bacteriological point of view in the study of infectious disease. Tuberculosis came to mean any infection caused by tubercle bacilli, whether or not tubercles could be found in the infected organs.

It is now obvious that the hereditary constitution, the physiological state, the nature of the environment and all the stresses and strains of life are of paramount importance in determining whether infection will manifest itself in the form of progressive disease. The "tubercular diathesis" of the old physicians was not such an empty concept after all. It has recovered its legitimate place among the "causes" of tuberculosis now that epidemiologists, physiologists, biochemists and immunologists have begun to define the mechanisms through which it affects susceptibility and resistance. Thus, it is likely that the present definition of the word "tuberculosis," based exclusively on the bacteriological causation of the disease, will become as outmoded as the word "consumption" became after 1830, and as the purely anatomical point of view became in 1882. Despite the efforts of purists, academies and dictionaries, definitions must evolve along with knowledge and concepts. The logic of words must always yield to the logic of the facts that they symbolize.

Part Three

CURE AND PREVENTION OF TUBERCULOSIS

CHAPTER X

The Evaluation of Therapeutic Procedures

LIKE MANY of his contemporaries, the famous English scientist, Thomas Young, had suffered from consumption during his early adulthood. But unlike most of the consumptives that he saw around him, he had made a full recovery. Being a physician as well as an experimental physicist, he decided that his personal experience entitled him to write *A Practical and Historical Treatise on Consumptive Diseases,* which was published in London in 1815. In his book, Young wisely emphasized the importance of early diagnosis, pointing out that general malaise, slight shortness of breath, cough even though not accompanied by pain, called for medical attention. He recommended as a diagnostic procedure the measurement of respiratory capacity by having the patient blow through a bent tube to displace water in an inverted jar, a technique now known as spirometry. He discussed the appearance of sputum in different diseases and described improvements over the methods in use since Hippocratic times to tell one type of sputum from another. He discussed the occurrence of consumption in different parts of the world and in different populations and presented some evidence suggesting its infectious nature.

In Young's book, side by side with so much shrewd medical thinking, there are found many of the old wives' tales that made the bulk of knowledge of tuberculosis at the beginning of the nineteenth century, particularly with reference to treatment. Like any ordinary man, this great investigator was fond of reporting cases of remarkable cures, and he was just as gullible as an untrained observer when evaluating the effects of remedies or treatments. It is worth mentioning in passing that most of the odd and now discredited therapeutic procedures of the past have been advocated by eminent representatives of medical science and practice. How can it be that experienced clinicians have erred just as widely as laymen in recommending methods of treatment that were found utterly useless in the course of time? The answer to this question lies in the fact that the course and final outcome of most diseases is unpredictable, being conditioned by the hereditary background of the patient, his past history, his psychic problems, his social environment, and countless other ill-defined factors.

The fatality of infectious maladies is not as great as is usually believed and, moreover, it changes to a remarkable degree with time. In the fifteenth and sixteenth centuries, for instance, syphilis behaved as a very acute infection in Europe, but by the eighteenth century its course had become milder and more chronic, a fair percentage of those afflicted with it recovering fully without treatment. Scarlet fever, pneumonia, measles, small pox, influenza are other examples, among many, of diseases which have fluctuated in severity during historical times and showed marked variations from one country to another. Obviously, then, clinical experience provides a sound basis of judgment only for a limited period of years and within a narrow range of environmental conditions.

The ethics of medical practice introduce still further difficulties in the evaluation of treatment. The more conscientious the physician, the more care he will take to place the patient under favorable conditions before introducing any new therapeutic measure. As a result, the natural vitality of the patient, helped by thoughtful and sympathetic attention, often performs the cure attributed to the new remedy. Moreover, the good physician instills into his patient his own hopes for recovery, creating mental peace and a confidence that are well-known to assist the body in overcoming disease. This important aspect of medical practice was tactfully brought out by Osler in a letter written to Dr. Pratt of Boston, who had sent him some papers describing the remarkable results he obtained with a new method for the treatment of a febrile active tuberculosis:

> The papers came this morning and I have read them with the keenest interest. I am afraid one element you have not laid proper stress upon — your own personality. Confidence and faith count for so much with these cases. The personal supervision and care is all important.

Trudeau, also, emphasized the influence of the doctor's personality on the well-being of the patient.

> . . . The doctor's . . . optimism is at once reflected to the patient and influences his condition accordingly. . . . In his hour of need the patient has no means of judging of the physician's intellectual attainments; it is the faith that radiates from the doctor's personality that he seizes upon and that is helpful to him. Any encouragement that emanates from the physician will help keep up the patient's courage and carry him through long days of illness and suffering to recovery. . . .

All the difficulties that stand in the way of the objective evaluation of therapeutic procedures are at their greatest in pulmonary tuberculosis, a chronic disease the course of which is affected by all sorts of obscure factors. This was the fact that Thomas Young had not recognized. He stated in his book that not one patient in a thousand recovered from phthisis without medical assistance and that the best possible care could, at the most, save the life of one in a hundred. His own recovery he regarded as almost miraculous. But even taking into consideration the fact that phthisis was then diagnosed late in its course, it is certain that in Young's time as now there were many patients with extensive pulmonary disease who lived a long life and not a few who recovered without treatment. In fact, Thomas Willis had voiced this opinion in 1684 in his *Practise of Physick.* Referring to patients with one or more ulcers or cavities in their lungs, he wrote: "Although they cast up much spittle and thick yellow matter every morning and sometimes all day, yet they live well enough in health, they breathe, eat and sleep well, are well in flesh or at least remain in an indifferent habit of body and frequently arrive at old age; in so much that some are said to have been consumptive thirty or forty years and have prolonged the disease even unto the term of their life (for that cause not being shortened)." Laënnec, who was a contemporary of Young, did believe that phthisis was often curable, even in the cavity stage.

Because of the uncertainty of its prognosis, tuberculosis has provided in the past — and remains today — the ideal disease for the promotion of ill-founded methods of treatment.[1] Before mentioning a few of the many cures which turned out to be mere illusions, and discussing those in favor today, it seems worth pointing out that, in general, methods for the treatment of disease can spring from two independent attitudes of mind. On the one hand, practical and thoughtful physicians have learned through experience a set of procedures which improve the well-being of their patients; they have also recognized by empirical observation the more or less specific curative effects of a few drugs on certain symptoms or diseases. Thus has slowly accumulated in the course of centuries a vast body of sound pragmatic knowledge still as valid and useful today as it ever was. Quinine, salicylic acid, digitalis, opiates and several other drugs have this honorable origin.

There has always existed, on the other hand, among both physicians and laymen, an urge to explain the mechanisms and manifestations of disease in the words of the prevalent scientific theories. And the temptation is always great to formulate methods of therapy that appear rational because they derive from logical considerations. Unfortunately, few are the cases where factual knowledge is sufficient to justify detailed scientific interpretations of disease, and to permit the use of rigorous logic in the practice of medicine. Yet very often the lure of logic has led to conclusions based on inadequate evidence and to practices more harmful than beneficial to the patient.

With his usual sagacity, Thomas Jefferson recognized the fallacies and dangers of medical practices based on pseudoscience:

> Having been so often a witness to the salutary efforts which nature makes to reestablish the disordered functions, he [the physician] should rather trust to their action than to hazard the interruption of that, and a greater derangement of the system, by conjectural experiments on a machine so complicated and so unknown as the human body, a subject so sacred as human life.
>
> But the adventurous physician goes on, and substitutes presumption for knowledge. From the scanty field of what is known, he launches into the boundless region of what is unknown. He establishes for his guide some fanciful theory of corpuscular attraction, of chemical agency, of mechanical powers, of stimuli, or irritability accumulated or exhausted, of depletion by the lancet and repletion by mercury, or some other ingenious dream, which lets him into all nature's secrets at short hand. On the principle which he thus assumes, he forms his table of nosology, arrays his diseases into families, and extends his curative treatment, by analogy, to all the cases he has thus arbitrarily marshalled together. I have lived myself to see the disciples of Hoffman, Boerhaave, Stahl, Cullen, Brown, succeed one another like the shifting figures of a magic lantern, and their fancies, like the dresses of the annual doll-babies from Paris, becoming, from their novelty, the vogue of the day, and yielding to the next novelty their ephemeral favor. The patient treated on the fashionable theory, sometimes gets well in spite of the medicine. . . .

Whether derived from empirical experience or from hypothetical considerations, methods of treatment do usually rule for a time with the authority of fashion. For, as Jefferson pointed out, physicians like other men are inclined either to follow uncritically the fads of their time, or to exhibit a misplaced independence of mind which leads them to deliberately promote theories of their own in opposition to those popular around them. Thus, medical practices are influenced directly or indirectly by the prevailing and fashionable scientific dogmas and by temperamental behavior. At the worst, these tendencies may lead to an attitude governed by gregariousness or by intellectual arrogance. But the human sympathy of the good physician usually helps him to ignore his pet theories and to overcome his prejudices. While longing to base his practice on scientific knowledge, he knows that the welfare of his patient is usually served better by the teachings of experience than by scientific dogma or philosophical beliefs. "To embrace all the relations and consequences of the most simple fact is not within the grasp of the human intellect," wrote Laënnec, "and the secrets of nature are more frequently betrayed to us by chance than extorted by the efforts of science."

It would be entertaining to write a history of the treatment of tuberculosis in the form of a procession of fads and counterfads each heralded by weighty theoretical preambles. The modern champions of outdoor life could be made to argue their thesis with illustrious physicians of a not distant past who feared above all the irritating effect of drafts and of night air. A place in the debate should be reserved for those who regarded the exhalations of cow houses as a sure remedy; no less a scientist than Joseph Priestley attributed the cure of his daughter to these fumes.[2] One could confront the various doctrines that have been formulated in the name of physiological principles to promote different types of climates and geographical situations: the seashore versus high mountains; the hot and dry deserts versus the cool Northern countries; the stimulation afforded by changing climate versus the relaxation that comes from a familiar environment.

Absolute immobility, in certain cases for periods of years, has received the sanction of modern physiological authorities, but several forms of physical exercise have also had their vogue: such as skiing, horseback riding continued for days at a time, and the involuntary motion of seasickness.[3] (Indeed, ingenious revolving chairs were once devised to provide tuberculous patients with an effective source of nausea.) To keep the lungs at rest is now the order of the day, and Thomas Beddoes also believed that those who play wind instruments are prone to phthisis. But Sax, the Belgian who invented the saxophone, came to the opposite conclusion half a century later and presented before the Paris Academy of Medicine a learned memoir claiming that the playing of wind instruments strengthens the lungs and should be used in the treatment of consumption.[4]

Nutrition, of course, is important. But, whereas some physicians thought it imperative to keep their patients on a starvation diet in order to combat fever, others wanted to correct emaciation by feeding twelve eggs daily, in addition to a rich, creamy diet. Fortunately, lobster and light wines have also had their partisans. Milk, it seems, has always been a specific for phthisis, but there were those who believed only in milk from goats pastured on high land and others who recommended human milk fed from the breast. As to asses' milk, it became so popular that Gideon Harvey, physician to the King of England, wondered whether "Ass-Patient or Ass-Doctor was the greater Ass." Needless to say, the same Gideon Harvey had his own secret remedy, a syrup probably containing millepedes.[5]

All the therapeutic errors of the past, and the controversies to which they gave rise, make it obvious that the evaluation of methods of treatment is fraught with great difficulty. It requires special methods which are complex and time-consuming, except in the case of the very few maladies where fatal outcome within a definite period of time is certain in the absence of therapy. Objective, convincing information concerning the effectiveness of many treatments of tuberculosis is still lacking. The conclusions now most commonly accepted have been reached on the basis of the clinical judgment of experienced physicians but, as already emphasized, experience gained at a certain time and under a certain set of conditions often becomes of doubtful value when circumstances change. Even during our lifetime there are not a few eminent clinicians, honored and respected teachers in great schools all over the world, who have made unjustified claims for the efficacy of procedures soon proved to be valueless. It is against this background of uncertainty that we shall now review the basis of some of the therapeutic practices now in honor, fully aware that ignorance, as well as personal and temporal prejudices, make this attempt a foolhardy venture.

CHAPTER XI

Treatment and Natural Resistance

As long as tuberculosis was diagnosed only in its late phase, the relief of distressing symptoms occupied the most important place in treatment. Many ancient procedures which have little or no effect on the course of the disease owe their lasting popularity to the fact that they improved the sense of well-being of the patient. To this class belong the inhalation of vapors from resinous, balsamic substances and emollient herbs, the sucking of cracked ice in hemoptysis, the use of opiates for quieting cough and the pains of intestinal tuberculosis.[1] Opium, as we have seen, enjoyed an immense vogue during the nineteenth century and was for a time considered as almost a specific for consumption. Even the skeptic, Pierre Louis, was much impressed by its beneficial effects. At the Hôpital de la Charité in Paris, Louis conducted the first objective tests to determine the effectiveness of different drugs, using sufficient numbers of patients to give statistical significance to his findings. He thus convinced himself that none of the drugs then known were of benefit in tuberculosis. But of opium he said, "It frequently produces so material an improvement in chronic phthisis, that the patients fancy themselves cured, or almost cured, after having taken a few doses."

Special mention must also be made of the use of cod-liver oil. Its first extensive clinical trials were carried out by Dr. C. J. Blasius Williams, one of the founders of the Brompton Hospital for Consumption, who introduced the new treatment there.

Strikingly beneficial effects were observed, particularly with regard to increasing the weight of the patients. In 1850, Williams stated in the *London Journal of Medicine* that "pure fresh Oil from the Livers of the Cod, is more beneficial in the treatment of Pulmonary Consumption than any agent, dietetic, or regimenal, that has yet been employed." Today, refined cod-liver oil is still widely employed to supplement the diet of the tuberculous patient in Vitamins A and D. Whether the cruder oil used in the past contained in addition some other beneficial factor as yet unidentified is a matter of conjecture.

Advanced tuberculosis being a wasting disease, the early physicians exercised much imagination to devise diets aimed at correcting the emaciation and increasing the strength of their patients. Historical and epidemiological evidence supports the clinical view that the individual's nutritional state is of paramount importance in tuberculosis, for there is no doubt that the disease is always more prevalent and more severe in areas or social situations where the diet is deficient in "high class" foods. It is also true that inadequate diet resulting from low economic status is usually accompanied by poor housing and crowding. There are a few cases where it seems possible to dissociate the effects of bad nutrition from those of unsanitary circumstances, often associated with poverty.

A few years ago a striking relation was observed between the diets and the physique and health of two African tribes, the Masai and Akikuyu, both of which live in a primitive state.[2] At the time of a survey made in 1931, the diet of the former tribe was found to consist chiefly of milk, raw blood and meat, whereas cereals supplemented with some roots and fruits were the only foods of the latter. Marked differences were found in the incidence of disease in the two tribes, pulmonary phthisis being many times more prevalent among the vegetarian Akikuyu than among the meat-eating Masai.

The course of tuberculosis in Denmark between 1914 and 1918

presents a case where lowered nutritional standards appear to have been the only or at least the preponderant factor in aggravating tuberculosis. The tuberculosis mortality in Denmark, which had been decreasing at a steady rate since 1900, showed a marked increase during the First World War between 1915 and 1917 but, curiously enough, the mortality curve resumed its downward trend before the end of the conflict. Denmark was not occupied during the First World War, did not take part in the fighting, and suffered no obvious social disturbance that could account for the increase in tuberculosis between 1915 and 1917. It is known, however, that enormous amounts of Danish meat and dairy products were exported to England during that period, and that the yearly consumption of meat per individual in Denmark fell sharply. After 1917 the submarine warfare interrupted the export trade, and it seems that the reversal of the trend in tuberculosis mortality occurred concomitantly with the return to more normal nutrition. (Appendix C.) There is some evidence that a similar situation occurred in certain parts of France during World War II. The consumption of meat and dairy products in Normandy and Brittany increased when difficulties of exchange interfered with the shipment of these foodstuffs to other parts of France. At the same time, the tuberculosis mortality decreased in these two provinces while it reached extremely high levels in Paris and many other cities, as well as in country districts with deficient food production. In England, statistical surveys have also revealed an astonishing correlation between consumption of "animal proteins" and tuberculosis mortality.

It must be emphasized again that, suggestive as they are, these correlations are not entirely convincing, since the decrease in availability of meat and dairy products usually coincides with other disturbances in the social fabric. Moreover, none of the observations made thus far are sufficiently precise to reveal the nature of the particular constituents of the food that affect resistance to tuberculosis.

It has been widely assumed that meat and dairy products act by virtue of their protein content, but it is equally plausible that they owe their beneficial effect to other unidentified dietary factors. Despite the countless pages that have been written concerning the relation of nutrition to tuberculosis, no knowledge whatever is available of the specific components of the diet that are involved, or of the mechanism by which the nutritional state modifies the course of disease. It is not even known whether foods that promote resistance act directly by affecting the tubercle bacilli or their toxins, or indirectly by increasing either the general physiological well-being or some specific defense and repair mechanism of the body. There have been a few timid attempts to determine the influence of *known* nutritional factors, particularly vitamins, on the course of infection; but the results have been equivocal. Indeed it is unlikely that this approach can ever yield the solution of the problem, for it would be surprising if the food components that cure nutritional deficiency diseases of noninfectious nature should prove also to be concerned in resistance to tuberculosis.

At the present time, one can conclude merely that poor nutrition is associated with increased susceptibility to tuberculosis, and that meat and dairy products appear rich in certain factors that increase resistance. But this is not enough to justify prescribing peculiar diets based on far-flung and unproven theories. In the absence of more precise knowledge, a variety of wholesome, nutritious and appetizing foods constitutes the best fare for the tuberculous patient.

The effect of climate, like that of nutrition, has been the subject of many unjustified fads. Old records provide ample evidence that in Europe and North America tuberculosis used to be far less frequent in the rural districts than in the large cities, as if there were something in "good air" that made for resistance to the disease. It is now known that the "bad" quality of the air in populated districts was in most cases the expression of a mode of living that greatly increased the chances of contact with virulent bacilli, rather than the result of noxious atmospheric gases. Today the tuberculosis mortality rate is lower in many large industrial cities than in farming areas, and country districts which were once essentially free of the disease became hotbeds of it at some later period.[3]

It will be recalled that Laënnec had found so few consumptive individuals in his native Brittany that he came to believe in some special virtue of the maritime air. And yet, the disease became rampant throughout Brittany a few decades after his death, probably on account of changes in living habits and of increased chances of infection caused by the greater facility of transportation. Similarly, it was long believed that the climate of Egypt was particularly helpful to the consumptive, but it is known that the present-day mortality from tuberculosis is extremely high in that country, although the Egyptian climate has not changed appreciably during historical times. Very precise information is available of the distribution of tuberculosis in Sweden during the past fifty years. Around 1900 the disease was almost unknown in the northern part of the country, though highly prevalent in the large cities in the more southern parts. Today the tuberculosis mortality rate in Stockholm is among the lowest in the world, whereas infection has been slowly increasing in the rural areas and islands farther north.

A book on *The Sanative Influence of Climate* was published in 1841 by Sir James Clark, the doctor who took care of Keats in Rome and later became physician to Queen Victoria. It presents detailed instructions for consumptives in the different phases of their disease, recommending sea voyages for early cases, mild equable climates for others, and making subtle distinctions as to weather between Rome or Nice, Pisa or Madeira. For patients who could not leave England he advised the use of self-regulating stoves permitting the constant control of temperature and recommended that windows be opened for only a few minutes each day.

The belief in the value of mild southern climates for the treatment of tuberculosis persisted throughout the nineteenth century, gaining support from the observation that people moving from southern to more northern regions were likely to contract fatal tuberculosis. Thus Rudolph Virchow pointed out that the inhabitants of Nubia became tuberculous when they moved into Egypt although Egypt was a health resort, and that tropical animals, especially monkeys, often died of tuberculosis when brought into Europe. Similarly, August Hirsch emphasized that persons moving from lower latitudes into colder regions usually became victims of scrofula, "all the more speedily and the more severely, the greater the difference between the climate of their new and of their old homes." The facts quoted by Virchow and by Hirsch were correct but their interpretation was erroneous. As the tropics were at the time still essentially free of tuberculosis, tropical men and animals were not exposed to infection in their native habitats. When they moved into Europe they suddenly came into contact with tuberculous individuals at a time when their own general resistance was probably decreased by the adaptation to life in a new environment. Exposure to infection under trying physiological conditions, and not some intrinsic deleterious effect of the northern climate, accounted for the severity of tuberculosis among them.

Today sanatoria are found on the seashore and in the high mountains, in the deserts of the Southwest and among the snows of the Adirondacks, remote in solitude and in the suburbs of the largest cities. Clearly the influence of the climate *per se* must not be very great, since such different locations have been found favorable for treatment. Nevertheless, it is generally held that a sunny and dry atmosphere is preferable for patients with catarrhal symptoms or for those suffering from laryngeal tuberculosis.[4] A region with a moderate altitude, free from mist, fogs, smoke and noxious vapors, with a fairly low humidity, mild temperatures oscillating between not too wide extremes, and with moderate air movements, would probably be considered as optimum for all types of tuberculosis. These conditions, of course, contribute to pleasant and easy living for almost anyone, and it is probable that the ideal climate for the treatment of tuberculosis would vary in detail from one individual to the other, depending upon physiological make-up, past experience and conditioning. The success of the Adirondacks as a health resort after the wilderness had become fashionable illustrates that the Southern lands are not necessarily the last refuge of the consumptive.

Although there exists as yet no precise information concerning the effects of climate, future research may throw unexpected light on the subject. The beneficial influence of heliotherapy and of ultraviolet rays in bone tuberculosis and, contrariwise, the toxic effects of excessive irradiation on the pulmonary tuberculous patient, demonstrate that lesions *can* respond favorably or unfavorably to physical factors of environment. Altitude must also have some influence, since it affects the composition and properties of the blood; in fact, it has been shown that the guinea pig, an animal originating in the high plateau of the Andes, is rendered more resistant to tuberculous infections when housed in chambers maintained at low atmospheric pressures simulating high elevation.

It is well possible that a clearer picture of the relation of climate to human tuberculosis could be obtained if techniques were available to study separately the effect of each of the components of climate. Since many independent factors of the physical environment act simultaneously to modify the response of the patient, the resultant effect is far too complex to be analyzed by observing the course of the disease in one location versus another. But the science of climate is yet unborn. Very little is known of the components of climate, and even less of the manner in which they affect the human machine in health and in disease.

Consumptives with fever, toxemia, and other obvious evidence of disease have always been advised to rest, to refrain as much as possible from speaking, and to achieve the tranquillity of mind that brings about relaxation of body and soul.[5] It is only during recent decades, however, that the rest treatment has also been applied to the less advanced stages of tuberculosis. Although the beneficial effects of rest are universally acknowledged, specialists differ somewhat as to the optimal manner of practising "rest." The differences in judgment are only of degree, not of principle; but they are brought into sharper relief by the knowledge that, in the past, physicians advocated some form of exercise in tuberculous conditions where absolute rest is now considered the most favorable policy.

Some of the past practices can be readily reconciled with modern points of view; long sea voyages, for example, provided the opportunity for many months of rest in the open air. By contrast, advocacy of horseback riding seems at first sight incompatible with present methods of treatment. Sydenham, the English Hippocrates of the eighteenth century, was so convinced of the value of riding that he considered it a specific remedy for tuberculosis.[6] "Bark (quinine)," he wrote, "is not surer cure for Ague than riding for phthisis." In the "Anecdota Sydenhamiana" the philosopher John Locke, who was also a physician and a friend and admirer of Sydenham's, tells how the famous doctor cured his nephew, who was suffering from phthisis.

> . . . Ye Doctor sent him into ye Count on Horseback (tho he was soe weak yt he could hardly walk), & ordered him to ride six or seven miles ye first day (which he did) & to encrease dayly his journey as he shd be able, until he had rid one hundred and fifty miles: When he had travelld half ye way his Diarrhoea stopt, & at last he came to ye end

> of his journey & was pretty well (at least somewhat better) & he had a good appetite: but when he had staid at his Sister's house some four or five days his Diarrhoea came on again; the Doctor had ordered him not to stay above two days at most; for if they stay before they are recovered this spoils all again; & therefore he betook himself to his riding again, and in four days he came up to London perfectly cured. The same course hath ye Doctor put others upon, especially in Pulmonick Diseases, & with ye like success when all things else had failed him; & he was not ashamed to own yt he was fain to borrow a cure from this way and now and then when he found himself pyzzled with some lingering Distemper nor reducible to a common and known disease.[7]

The regimen on which Sydenham put his nephew would constitute a painful physical ordeal for most modern men. But it must be remembered that horseback riding was then the most widely used form of transportation and the easiest way to be carried about without much effort. Benjamin Marten's advice to consumptive persons a century later leaves no doubt that, according to his judgment, the mildest possible form of exercise was "riding on Horseback in the manner of Travellers and not furiously."

> And the best Method that I know of, which even People who have continued Business in Town may comply with, is to have their Families in the Country at about eight or ten miles from London and constantly go thither in the Evening and return to Town early every Morning. . . . Their Minds, also, will be much better entertained while they are on Horseback this way, which is a kind of Business, than if they were riding out to take the Air.

Riding in one form or another remained in honor as a method of treatment long after Sydenham. In Holland, the physiologist Van Swieten recommended that patients of the lower classes who were confined to sedentary occupations endeavor to find employment as coachmen. In America, Benjamin Rush told of a cobbler who abandoned his awl and became a coachman on the advice of his physician. He was well as long as he remained in the saddle but lost his health when he returned to cobbling. In a paper read before the American Climatological Association in 1889 Bowditch narrated a similar experience. In 1808, at the age of thirty-five, his father had suffered from severe pulmonary tuberculosis. After the acute symptoms had subsided, he began a drive of several weeks with a friend through New England in an open buggy. The elder Bowditch recovered from his disease, and when he died at the age of sixty-seven from cancer of the stomach, a healed lesion was found in his lungs at autopsy.

In all ages, physicians have also been preoccupied with the importance of securing for the consumptive an environment where not only the body but also the mind is free from unessential efforts.[8] Richard Morton had urged that "the patient by all Lawful ways industrially lay aside care, melancholy and all poring of his Thoughts as much as ever he can and endeavor to be cheerful." And, in a similar vein, Marten expressed his concern that the mental restlessness which plagues the life of those made idle by tuberculous disease might nullify the good effects of rest at home. "When People labouring under this Distemper are continuously sitting still, musing on and lamenting on their own sickly condition and constantly confine themselves to their Houses and Chambers . . . , they take a ready means to promote the Distemper instead of their own Health."

Thus, it is clear that the old physicians were as eager as are the modern specialists to secure physical and mental rest for their patients. They did their best to find a formula of relaxation compatible with the habits and facilities of their social environment. Horseback riding may well have been at that time the most comfortable and relaxing manner to sit in the open air, while prolonged residence in dark, smelly and stuffy chambers was probably conducive to physical and mental fretfulness rather than to rest. The controversies concerning the extent and thoroughness with which rest should be practised by tuberculous patients originate from deficiencies in physiological knowledge. The words "rest" and "fatigue," which appear so simple and straightforward, convey in reality ill-defined concepts colored by habits and emotions. Until they are defined in terms of more precise understanding, and until techniques are available for measuring and controlling true physiological rest, physicians will have to use empirical experience and their judgment of human nature in order to devise for each individual the best regimen for optimal repose.

It was clinical experience that revealed the therapeutic effects of healthy living, good food and rest in tuberculosis. But it took the resources of physiological, pathological, bacteriological and chemical sciences to bring about the more active forms of treatment, such as pulmonary collapse, surgery and the use of antimicrobial drugs.

As early as 1696 Baglivi had reported in Italy cases of soldiers who had recovered from phthisis after having received deep wounds in the chest. This original observation had impressed a physician of Liverpool, James Carson, who wrote in 1822, "The cure, both of the wound and of the previous disease depended upon the same cause, the reduction of the diseased and the wounded lung to a state of collapse."

Carson opened the thoracic cavity of rabbits and became convinced that "one of the lungs of an animal may be reduced to a state of collapse without the other being affected." This suggested to him that it might be possible to treat some pulmonary diseases, consumption in particular, by opening the chest on the side of the diseased lung, and thus allowing it to collapse by virtue of its own elasticity. The first patient that he treated by this method of artificial pneumothorax was a merchant of Liverpool whose four brothers had died of phthisis a few years before. The operation was done at the patient's own request.

> An incision calculated to admit air freely into the chest was made between the sixth and seventh ribs. As the sound usually heard upon the opening being made into the chest and produced, no doubt, by the rapid passage of air through the opening, was not perceived in this case it was suspected that the lung did not collapse and that the adhesion prevented the entrance of air. It was not deemed advisable to make a further examination at the time.

As Carson suspected, it is probable that his patient's disease was too advanced and complicated by adhesions to give the operation any chance of success. Moreover, Carson's operative technique was crude, consisting merely in making an incision into the thorax and allowing as much air to enter as was pulled in by the collapse of the lung; a new opening in the chest wall had to be made for each refill. Because of these difficulties and despite further sporadic attempts, the method was soon abandoned, and Carson's name and work were forgotten.

In 1882 (the year of the discovery of the tubercle bacillus), the distinguished Italian, Carlo Forlanini, again suggested that pulmonary phthisis could be treated by establishing artificial pneumothorax through the chest wall. Furthermore, he had the idea of introducing nitrogen by means of a large hypodermic needle, a convenient technique that permitted frequent refills. Although his results were at first meager, Forlanini persisted and after a few years was in a position to report a number of successful cases that convinced medical opinion. Once the principle of treatment by artificial pneumothorax was accepted, efforts were made all over the world to achieve collapse of the diseased lung by other techniques, in particular thoracoplasty and pneumoperitoneum.[9]

Collapse therapy is possible only because man can carry on fairly normal activities even when deprived of much of his lung tissue for a more or less prolonged period of time. This fact suggested the possibility that certain forms of pulmonary disease might be treated by surgical removal of the affected lobe, but the operation was long considered so dangerous as to discourage even the boldest surgeons. It was an accidental observation that revealed the potential usefulness of thoracic surgery in tuberculosis. In the course of surgical treatment of diseases erroneously diagnosed as bronchial carcinomas, tuberculous lungs were removed by error on several occasions, the correct diagnosis being made only after the operation. Some of the patients so treated did well, and their recovery gave impetus to the surgical resection of tuberculous lung tissue.

The marvelous development of surgical techniques during recent years, facilitated by the availability of antimicrobial drugs, has increased enormously the safety of thoracic surgery and appears to give a wide field to this form of therapy.

Surgical operations on tuberculous lungs, joints, kidneys and nodes permit the removal of the obvious foci of disease. Even when the infection appears localized in only one organ, however, tubercle bacilli are usually present in other parts of the body. Thus, complete recovery from the disease depends upon the ability of the normal defense mechanisms to hold in check the bacilli not removed by surgical intervention. Similarly, collapse measures aim at interrupting the progress of the infection in a badly diseased part of the lung in the hope that physiological and immune processes will prevent further spreads to other areas of the body. The mechanisms by which collapse interferes with the progress of infection are unknown, although the effect is commonly explained away by the statement that the collapsed lung is put at rest because it is immobilized. In addition to this purely mechanical immobilization, however, collapse brings about profound physiological changes that modify in a complex manner the behavior of tissue cells and interfere with the multiplication of the bacilli. But there is no basis on which to judge which of these effects is significant in deciding the outcome of the infective process.

While "rest" is always emphasized as the most important aspect of the treatment of tuberculosis, it must be noted that the word is used promiscuously to express a whole range of meanings extending from obvious physical concepts to the most subtle psychic influences. There is no clear indication that *putting the lung at rest* by pulmonary collapse has the same physiological effects as the practice of strict *bed rest,* or that either of these forms of treatment bears any relation to the *mental rest* achieved by freedom from worry and from painful emotions. No one knows how these different types of rest bring about their therapeutic results, whether they favor the healing process around lesions already established, or increase resistance to the invasion of areas of the body as yet unaffected. In fact, it is probable that in general successful control of the disease demands some positive action on the part of the tissues, rather than the passive cessation of physical activity which is implied by rest.

But, whatever the mechanisms of the beneficial effects, rest there must be — mechanical, physiological and psychological.

The use of the word "rest" in so many different connotations symbolizes the belief that resistance to tuberculosis is determined by factors of the host that can be influenced by the proper way of life. Although the different aspects of rest may each influence the response of the patient to infection by means of unrelated processes, it is also possible that they all operate indirectly through one or a very few common mechanisms — for example, through the hormones which control tissue reactions. Recent studies on the dramatic effects exerted by the components of the adrenal-anterior pituitary system (ACTH and cortisone) on the course of tuberculosis illustrate how physical and mental stresses can have indirect but far-reaching effects on infectious disease.

Some principles, at least, appear well established. The body can oppose tuberculous infection with effective means of resistance which are rarely overcome. Some mismanagement of the human machine must occur before the bacilli succeed in gaining a permanent foothold and in causing extensive ravages. It is an almost constant clinical experience that patients with recently discovered active tuberculosis have undergone excessive physical or mental exertion. Even after infection has become established, the progress of the disease is usually arrested if the natural defense mechanisms of the body are given a chance to reassert themselves. At the present time, it is only by empirical procedures that the physician can intervene to put these defense mechanisms back in operation. His task would be much facilitated, and his intervention more effective, if precise knowledge were available of the physiological processes that interfere with the multiplication of tubercle bacilli and with the manifestation of their toxic effects.

CHAPTER XII

Drugs, Vaccines and Public Health Measures

THE GERM THEORY opened several new lines of attack against tuberculosis. It stimulated the search for antimicrobial drugs useful in treatment, and for vaccines capable of immunizing the well person against infection. It led to the development of techniques for the detection of infected individuals and to sanitary measures for preventing the spread of disease. The germ theory thus made it appear possible to break the chain of infection and to eradicate tuberculosis from human societies. Although much progress towards these goals has been made during the seventy years that have elapsed since Koch's discovery, unforeseen and formidable obstacles have been encountered on the way.

Tubercle bacilli are not as "tough" as their reputation claims, and, contrary to general belief, there exist many types of substances capable of inhibiting their growth, or of causing their rapid death in the test tube. But, as is the case with other microorganisms, most of these substances are ineffective in the body. The first convincing reports of therapeutic effect in tuberculosis of the guinea pig were published in the 1930's – first with sulfanilamide and then with diamino-diphenyl-sulfone. Although these two drugs proved useless in the treatment of human tuberculosis, the demonstration of their effectiveness in animals acted as a great stimulus for further research and soon led to the discovery of several substances which can be used in man. Of these, streptomycin and para-amino-salicylic acid (PAS) appear, to date, the most useful; they exhibit an immense activity against tubercle bacilli both in the test tube and in the body, and are relatively nontoxic. Both exert in a large percentage of cases a striking beneficial effect on the course of tuberculosis in the lungs and in other organs. Most spectacular was the demonstration that streptomycin could save from death a number of patients suffering from miliary and meningeal tuberculosis, two forms of the disease that were almost invariably fatal before the use of this drug.

Unfortunately, streptomycin and PAS rarely bring about a permanent and complete cure of pulmonary tuberculosis, even when they initially cause a dramatic arrest of the spread of the disease. Study of this disturbing fact soon revealed that the bacilli often become resistant to the drugs, in particular to streptomycin, after a few weeks to a few months of treatment.[1] This change of properties of the bacilli is certainly responsible for many therapeutic failures, but development of drug resistance is only one part of the story. A more difficult and more important aspect of the problem is the fact that tuberculosis presents peculiar characteristics that render it less amenable to drug treatment than are other infectious diseases.

Tubercle bacilli, it will be recalled, are readily engulfed by tissue cells and can live for prolonged periods of time within them. The intracellular environment constitutes a shelter which affords them a partial protection against the antimicrobial drugs present in the body fluids. Furthermore, tuberculosis results in the death of large masses of tissue, which persist in the form of caseous material. Since it is almost certain that the drugs are much less effective in the presence of dead tissue, they are therefore poorly able to cause injury to the bacilli surviving in caseous areas. Thus, the problem of the chemotherapy of tuberculosis is not merely one of finding a more "powerful" nontoxic substance capable of inhibiting the growth of tubercle bacilli or killing them. Its complete solution demands that some way be found to deal with the bacilli in the peculiar protective environments that the tissues provide for them. Investigation of this problem is complicated by the fact that tuberculosis in man evolves in a manner different from that observed in animals; it is difficult in particular to produce experimentally the type of pulmonary phthisis with caseation and cavitation. For this reason, many new therapeutic procedures which are effective in the tuberculosis of guinea pigs or mice prove of little or no use in the human disease. As this book goes to press, a new drug – isonicotinic acid hydrazide – is being introduced for the treatment of human tuberculosis and heralded as potentially capable of eradicating the disease. May it live up to its promises and render this chapter obsolete.*

The demonstration that tuberculosis is caused by a living microorganism gave ground immediately for the hope that it would be possible to develop a protective vaccine against it. In

* Unfortunately, the "miracle" drug which made for such exciting headlines and photographs, in the press of mid-February 1952, will probably be regarded as just another treatment when re-evaluated in the light of experienced judgment. There is no doubt that isonicotinic acid hydrazide is immensely active against tubercle bacilli, and can arrest within a few days certain forms of *acute* tuberculosis. These acute conditions, being often rapidly fatal when left untreated, create the atmosphere in which any drug preventing death is hailed as miraculous. But, however dramatic in its course, acute tuberculosis constitutes only a minor part of the total problem. It is by causing *chronic* pulmonary disease that tubercle bacilli impose on society such a heavy burden of suffering and protracted death. And the control of this chronic disease is the real touchstone of antituberculosis measures.

There is as yet no evidence that the new drugs have satisfied this exacting criterion. In fact, the bacilli lodged in old lesions do not appear to be any more readily affected by these drugs than they are by streptomycin and PAS. Since most tuberculous disease is recognized only when the lesions are already well established, the problem of eradication of tuberculosis from society is not likely to be solved by the use of any drug, however powerful and nontoxic. Tuberculosis will be conquered only when man has learned to function according to a physiological way of living that renders him more resistant to tubercle bacilli, and when he has created a social environment that protects him from exposure to infection.

fact, it took but a few years to find that one can establish by various methods of vaccination a low but significant level of antituberculous immunity. But, despite countless studies in experimental animals and in man for several decades, it has not yet been possible to go much beyond these early results, and the vaccinated individual cannot be given a reasonable assurance that he is safe from progressive tuberculous disease.

Large numbers of recipes have been proposed for the preparation of vaccines, from almost every known species of tubercle-like bacilli, virulent or avirulent, alive or killed by a variety of treatments, intact or extracted by acids, alkalis, or organic solvents. For each vaccine there are on record enthusiastic claims of protective action, and also accounts of complete failure. All these conflicting reports could be used to discredit the validity of "scientific" evidence, or at least of what is too often published under the guise of evidence in scientific journals. But the controversies also serve a more useful purpose. They teach the student of tuberculosis that a few surviving guinea pigs do not constitute proof for the effectiveness of the treatment that the animals have received, and that statistics are often a will-of-the-wisp which lure their eager followers into the marshy lands of indecisive experimentation.

For the sake of convenience, it seems best to disregard chronological order in the development of studies on vaccination, and to list in a schematic manner the different types of vaccines which have survived to date.

It is known that a certain degree of immunity can be elicited by injecting into experimental animals bacilli killed by heat or by antiseptics.[2] Although this method of vaccination has been used with encouraging results in human beings, it has few advocates at the present time. The occurrence of unpleasant abscesses at the site of injection, and the fear that the immunity induced is of a low order and evanescent, have militated against its adoption. It is likely, however, that further studies could lead to the development of more effective and less toxic "killed vaccines."

Many attempts have been made to produce immunity by using for vaccination living bacilli totally devoid of virulence for man. A culture isolated from a water turtle was widely promoted for this purpose under the name of "Friedman vaccine" half a century ago. Although all evidence shows that it has no anti-tuberculous activity whatever, it is still being produced commercially in several parts of the world. So vigorous is the life instilled into useless medicines by human hopes and gullibility!

The intense interest in vaccination at the turn of the nineteenth century emboldened some physicians in Europe and North America to inject very small amounts of virulent bacilli into a few human beings, in the hope of producing thereby an abortive disease that would elicit immunity. Fortunately this dangerous practice was soon abandoned. A more conservative and fruitful approach was proposed in 1889 by Maffucci in Italy. Taking advantage of the low virulence of human bacilli for the bovine species, he suggested that cattle could be safely vaccinated with living cultures of these microorganisms. Modifications of his method were for a time utilized with some measure of success particularly for the vaccination of calves, and Robert Koch himself published experiments that had favorable results. Shortly after 1900 von Behring in Germany went as far as prognosticating that bovine tuberculosis could be eradicated from the world by the use of his "Bovo Vaccine." It was soon recognized, however, that although human bacilli do not cause progressive and fatal disease in cows, they survive for months or years in their bodies and may appear in a viable form in the milk. The method was therefore abandoned completely because of its potential danger for human health.

A safer application of the same principle has been recently tested in England with the type of tubercle bacilli that causes disease in voles. The vole bacilli are not virulent for guinea pigs and cattle and elicit in these animals resistance to infection. It is probable that they could also serve as a vaccine in man, but their use presents difficulties similar to those that have been encountered in BCG vaccination, which will be discussed later in this chapter.

The method of vaccination most widely in use at the present time is based upon a principle discovered by Pasteur in 1882, namely the injection of "attenuated" forms of virulent bacilli. It has long been known that, like other pathogenic microorganisms, virulent tubercle bacilli can undergo hereditary modifications, resulting in the loss of their ability to cause progressive disease. Despite this decrease in virulence, the "attenuated" bacilli remain capable of multiplying to a certain extent in the human and animal body, producing a mild self-limited disease which so modifies the infected individual as to increase his resistance to a subsequent fully virulent infection.

The possibility of vaccinating with attenuated cultures of tubercle bacilli had been recognized very early, in particular by the pioneer American investigator Trudeau. Working in his small, primitive laboratory in the isolated village of Saranac Lake, he carefully compared the different types of vaccine then available and reached conclusions to which little, if anything, of importance has been added during recent years. It is of historical interest to present in Trudeau's own words the digest of his experience that he presented in 1905.

> Dead tubercle bacilli increase, though to a very slight degree, the animal's resistance to subsequent inoculation.
>
> The living attenuated bacillus gives a stronger degree of immunity than the same bacillus killed by heat.
>
> The degree of attenuation of the bacillus used as vaccine bears a distinct relation to the degree of protection it affords in guinea pigs to subsequent inoculation with virulent human cultures. A culture still capable of producing a very small amount of cell destruction, and of spreading to the neighboring inguinal nodes, gives better protection than

> one which produces hardly any appreciable and purely localized tissue changes.
>
> Cultures derived from cold-blooded animals and which only grow at room temperature, have brought about no appreciable degree of immunity.[3]

By far the most extensive studies of antituberculosis vaccination have been carried out with the famous strain BCG (Bacillus Calmette Guérin). When first isolated from a case of tuberculosis in cattle, this culture was highly virulent for many types of animals and most probably for man, but it became progressively attenuated while being cultivated in the test tube by the French bacteriologists Calmette and Guérin. In a long series of painstaking studies carried out at the Pasteur Institute in Lille, and then in Paris, these investigators established that BCG had lost its ability to cause progressive fatal disease in cattle, guinea pigs, rabbits and monkeys, but could still increase the resistance of these animals to virulent infection. Countless experiments, performed all over the world, under all sorts of conditions, and in several animal species, have confirmed beyond any doubt this loss of virulence and the retention of immunizing power.

Injection of BCG produces in animals a very mild disease consisting of the dissemination and multiplication of the bacilli in the different organs, with production of small tubercles. Within a very few weeks, however, the bacilli stop multiplying, although they survive in the tissues for an indefinite period of time. The lesions do not spread, but instead disappear slowly. This self-limited infection induces a state of partial resistance which may last several years, and which is effective against virulent bacilli of both human and bovine origin. It must be emphasized, however, that immunity is never absolute, and that guinea pigs, however much vaccine they have received, eventually succumb to virulent infection, although more slowly than do the nonvaccinated animals. Present evidence strongly suggests that vaccination with BCG does not prevent the establishment of the virulent bacilli, but only retards their spread. The same observations apply to vaccination with vole bacilli.

Once convinced of the safety and immunizing power of BCG in animals, Calmette and his collaborators undertook a large program of vaccination of children born in tuberculous families. At first, the vaccine was administered by mouth and only to newborn babies. As it often failed to "take" under these conditions, Swedish workers recommended injecting it *beneath* the skin and thus succeeded in eliciting a positive tuberculin state in most of the children and adults whom they vaccinated. Unfortunately, draining abscesses developed so frequently at the site of the injection and in the regional lymph nodes that the subcutaneous route had to be abandoned. The method most commonly used at the present time consists in injecting the vaccine *into* the superficial layers of the skin or depositing a drop of it on the skin and pricking with a sharp needle as is done in vaccination against smallpox. The local lesions are usually mild and heal in a few weeks; draining sinuses from local lymph nodes are rare.

BCG causes in man a mild infection probably very similar to that produced in experimental animals and it can also induce a level of relative immunity of the same order. The vaccine possesses, therefore, many desirable attributes. Yet, although it has been available and used for some thirty years, controversies are still raging concerning its place in antituberculosis control.

The fact that BCG originated from a virulent culture was the cause of great fears concerning its safety some two decades ago. It is true that the experience gained with other microbial species makes it theoretically probable that one could bring about a reversal of BCG to full virulence by the proper laboratory artifices, but this has never been found to occur under ordinary circumstances. Enormous amounts of vaccine have been injected into the most susceptible animals, and also in man, without causing progressive tuberculous disease or the appearance of virulent bacillary forms, and it seems certain that the proper degree of attenuation of the culture can be maintained by adequate techniques.

The Lübeck tragedy did much to increase the fears attending the use of the vaccine. The newborn babies who developed tuberculosis had just been vaccinated with a preparation labeled BCG, and the suspicion naturally arose that the microorganisms had undergone a change of properties in the unfortunate children. Although a commission of eminent German experts established beyond doubt that what had been distributed as BCG was in reality a culture of virulent bacilli, the accident left a deep scar in the popular and medical mind and discouraged the practice of vaccination for a number of years. The error emphasized the technical difficulties involved in the use of vaccines made up of living organisms. Both in the case of BCG and of the vole bacilli, present methods of preparation and distribution make it necessary to utilize the vaccines within a few days after their preparation. This short period of time does not allow the performance of the safety tests considered essential for all other types of biological products employed in human medicine.

The objections to the use of BCG and the vole bacilli based on potential danger of the vaccines arise from technical difficulties which can and certainly will be solved. Of more fundamental importance are other problems for which no practical solution is yet in sight. In many countries the tuberculin test has become a specific and often dependable tool for the early diagnosis of infection, particularly in children, and for the detection of spreaders of bacilli. As BCG, and the vole bacilli as well, produce in man a state of allergy to tuberculin which can hardly be differentiated from that caused by real tuberculosis, vaccination deprives the physician and public health officer of one of the most effective means of diagnosis. This would be of little consequence if vaccination gave promise of eradicating tuberculosis completely, but the vaccines now available are not sufficiently effective to justify such hope.

There are many physicians, in fact, who believe that the degree of immunity afforded by vaccination is far too low to be of practical significance for the protection of human beings living in civilized communities, or even of cattle under field conditions. While several controlled trials have revealed a protective effect of the vaccine, a few others have given disappointing results. The very existence of conflicting claims and of long-lasting controversies points to many unsolved problems.

It is certain that immunity develops only if the attenuated bacilli multiply in the tissues of the vaccinated individual. On the other hand, this multiplication must be kept within well-limited bounds in order to prevent the occurrence at the site of injection of abscesses which, although entailing no real danger, are somewhat alarming to the patient and to his family. The practice of vaccination demands, therefore, a most skillful control of all the factors affecting the extent of bacillary multiplication in man. And these factors are many. They include the number of living bacilli injected, the degree of attenuation of their virulence, the technique of injection, the physiologic state of the vaccinated individual, and whether or not this individual has ever before been in contact with tubercle bacilli. Unfortunately, accurate knowledge is lacking with regard to most of these aspects of the problem. Very properly, the greatest emphasis is always placed on administering the vaccine in such a manner that no unpleasant reaction ensues, but because vaccination must be safe for all, it is probably ineffective for many, and the degree of effectiveness is, at the present time, unpredictable and unmeasurable.

Even after the technical problems concerning the procedures of vaccination have been completely solved, it may long remain difficult to define its place in antituberculosis campaigns. The countries where tuberculosis is the most prevalent are also those where the practice of vaccination will present the greatest difficulties. To be effective, vaccines must be administered before infection with virulent bacilli has taken place, and for this reason, ideally, children should be removed from their tuberculous environment, usually from their own family, until immunity has been established. The social problems involved in this step are the greater the less fortunate the economic situation of the family, and it is precisely in these low income groups that the chances of infection are the greatest. Moreover, the practice of vaccination by the methods now available requires great technical and administrative skill, while the medical and public health services are often handicapped by inadequate funds and staff in poor countries with a high tuberculosis rate.

To the uninitiated, it may appear that the most direct way to pass judgment on vaccination is to observe its effects in the places where it has been widely practised. In reality, this is an extremely complex if not an impossible task. A few examples may be in order to illustrate the difficulties encountered.

Tuberculosis mortality rates have decreased at a most gratifying rate in Denmark, Norway and Sweden, countries which have been very active in the scientific and practical use of BCG. Nowhere, however, has the decrease been more spectacular than in Iceland, where mortality fell from 203 per 100,000 population in 1929 to 26 in 1949 although neither BCG nor any other immunizing agent was used! In the state of Minnesota, with a population predominantly Scandinavian in origin, tuberculosis mortality rate was 107 per 100,000 in 1916; it was 13.6 in 1949, one of the lowest in the world, lower than the rate of 19 prevailing in Denmark at the same time. Minnesota is conquering the disease without resorting to vaccination.

Tuberculosis has long been known to be very prevalent in Japan, and became a particularly alarming problem at the end of World War II. To meet the emergency, the Japanese authorities instituted a vast program of vaccination with BCG soon after the end of the conflict. The tuberculosis mortality in Japan fell from 280 per 100,000 in 1945 to 181 in 1948. However, this does not prove that BCG played any significant part in the control of the disease, for experience has repeatedly shown that tuberculosis increases during wars and revolutions and recedes equally rapidly when social conditions return to normal. (Appendix C.)

Thus, it appears unlikely that the practical value of vaccination can be determined from changes in the prevalence and severity of tuberculosis in a given country. Two other courses of action appear possible for investigating the problem. One would be to select a large population sufficiently stable to be followed for a number of years, vaccinate half of its individuals taken at random, leave the other half unvaccinated, and follow the comparative incidence of tuberculosis in the two groups. Although simple in appearance, this test presents formidable administrative difficulties and could be properly carried out only by well endowed and highly sophisticated public health services. It has not yet been put into operation on an adequate scale anywhere.

The other approach is more limited in scope and in significance, but is somewhat easier to conduct. It consists in studying the effect of vaccination in small and well-defined groups of individuals in whom tuberculosis is a special danger because of their mode of life or professional activities. Although tuberculosis is an important problem in some of the mining industries, miners cannot be considered for such a study, because silicosis is common among them and because recent findings show that attenuated bacilli can cause progressive and fatal disease in silicotic animals.

Most observations made on groups of medical students, nurses and babies vaccinated with BCG have revealed an unusually low incidence of tuberculosis, thus providing evidence in favor of vaccination. In these special and limited studies, the vaccinated individuals receive at the same time as the vaccine the benefit of the most enlightened practices designed to protect them in every possible manner; children are separated from their tuberculous parents, students and nurses are warned against the dangers of infection and of strenuous living. Thus, the higher the ethics and experience of the physician in charge of the vaccination experiment, the more difficult it is to dissociate the protective effects of vaccination from those of the other medical practices that he feels duty-bound to introduce in the test. Granted all these difficulties of experimentation with human beings, it appears nevertheless certain that the protective effect of BCG vaccination has been established in a few well-controlled tests on a small scale.[4]

Even when practiced under ideal conditions, however, vaccination never succeeds in completely preventing tuberculosis in the vaccinated group. Moreover, the duration of the immunity that it affords is still uncertain. Thus, much remains to be learned before it is known under what special circumstances vaccination can prove of benefit. The prevalence of tuberculosis in the area under consideration; the rate of progress in its control by sanitation, and other public health measures; the social and economic status of the community — all these are as important as the bacteriological aspects of the problem in defining the place of vaccination in antituberculosis campaigns.

Needless to say, all these uncertainties weigh little against the eagerness of those who feel that any promising technique must be used to check the spread of tuberculosis in the destitute parts of the world. Immediately after the war, teams of Scandinavian doctors, financed at first by the Danish Red Cross, began a campaign of vaccination of children in Central Europe. In 1948 the United Nations International Children's Emergency Fund made an agreement with the Swedish and Danish Red Cross and the "Norwegian Help for Europe" to extend the campaign to the rest of the world. Under the technical guidance of the World Health

Organization, the program is now moving forward under the name of "Joint Enterprise." Whole populations are being skin-tested in an effort to detect the individuals who are tuberculin-negative and therefore presumed to be in need of vaccination. More than twenty-five million persons have already been vaccinated in this greatest mass immunization in history. Moreover, the Scandinavian doctors and nurses are organizing direct demonstration clinics to help train local workers who will carry on the program.

For reasons already discussed, it will probably never be possible to determine the effects of the Joint Enterprise on the course of tuberculosis in the countries where it operates. It is certain that the disease will not be eradicated by vaccination, and it is likely that tuberculosis will remain a grave problem even in vaccinated populations if economic difficulties and social disturbances continue to interfere with general well-being. But if peace returns and hope flourishes again in the hearts of men, tuberculosis will recede as it has always done, spontaneously, when life has become easier and happier. And then it will make little difference whether vaccination, or merely better food, brighter lodgings, cleaner environment and gladness of heart have been responsible for the control of tuberculosis. BCG will deserve its share of the credit as a symbol of those generous impulses which help to create a better world.

The recent years have seen much increased interest in the study of immunity, and new discoveries will eventually throw light on a number of perplexing questions. In the meantime, any attempt at summarizing present knowledge is necessarily colored by individual prejudices and specialized knowledge or ignorance. There is universal agreement that vaccination with attenuated cultures can increase resistance to tuberculous infection, but the protection that it affords is of a low order. The method used for the preparation of the vaccines is primitive, and the techniques for the evaluation of their protective power practically nonexistent. Vaccination will prove most difficult to carry out in an effective manner in the countries and social groups where tuberculosis is most widespread, and it is unlikely that its practice on a large scale is justified in places where the disease is rapidly decreasing. With the techniques presently available, vaccination may prove most useful in certain groups having an unusually high degree of exposure to tuberculous disease, provided contraindications such as silicosis or malnutrition have been ruled out. This estimate of the usefulness of vaccination is not as sanguine as that made by its ardent advocates, but it is sufficient to make of Calmette and Guérin's work one of the landmarks on the road to the conquest of tuberculosis.

Whereas the final place of vaccination in antituberculosis programs is still unsettled, it is certain that its scientific study has focused attention upon one of the most important problems of tuberculosis, that of immunity. There is no longer any doubt that resistance can be increased by artificial procedures, and there is no apparent reason why the injection of *living* bacilli should be the most effective way to elicit this resistant state. It will certainly be possible to obtain in a purified form some substance capable of eliciting immunity, and to use it for vaccination in lieu of the living attenuated tubercle bacilli. When this objective has been achieved, it will become easier to control the process of vaccination and, perhaps, to attain more dependable and higher levels of immunity with less danger of objectionable reactions. In the case of all infectious diseases, the use of living cultures of the infectious agent is only the first step in the development of immunizing procedures. Pasteur himself, who discovered the immunizing power of attenuated cultures, clearly stated a few years later that the future was in the use of lifeless extracts, of what he called "chemical vaccines." It would be most surprising if a vaccine prepared in 1920 on the basis of principles worked out in 1882 should be the final formula for immunization against tuberculosis.

It is probable that the most important contribution of bacteriological science to the control of tuberculosis has been in guiding efforts to prevent the spread of tubercle bacilli. The effects of prevention far outweigh those of treatment and vaccination. It is by preventive measures that bovine tuberculosis has been practically wiped out in certain parts of the world, and this achievement has had far-reaching consequences for the control of the human disease.[5] Wherever it has been achieved, the eradication of tuberculosis from cattle has brought about the almost complete disappearance of human infection caused by bacilli of the bovine type.[6] It has helped to lower the cost of production of meat and dairy products, and has led indirectly thereby to an improvement of human nutrition and higher resistance to infection. Moreover, the fact that tuberculosis has been eradicated from certain animal populations has fostered the confidence that it could also be eradicated from human populations.

In the United States, the eradication of bovine tuberculosis was carried out by the drastic and costly policy of slaughtering all tuberculous animals. Over 8 per cent of the cattle were found infected when the program was begun in 1917. From that time until 1941, more than two hundred million animals were tested with tuberculin in order to detect the carriers of infection. All those found tuberculin-positive, and therefore likely to be infected, were slaughtered. At the present time less than 0.5 per cent of the cattle are still reactors, and there is reason to believe that many of these are not tuberculous.[7]

Bovine tuberculosis has also been eradicated more or less completely from Finland, the Channel Isles, Denmark, Sweden and Norway. In these European countries, however, eradication has been achieved without resorting to wholesale slaughtering. Animals found positive to tuberculin were removed from contact with the noninfected, and in particular from the newborn calves. The reactors with only little disease were kept for milk and meat production, thus minimizing economic losses. The non-reactors were used for the raising of animals free of tuberculosis. By a skillful policy of segregation, it proved possible to develop "accredited" herds in a remarkably short time and at relatively little cost.

Although the policy of segregation cannot be applied to human beings as ruthlessly as it has been to cattle, modern societies are coming to the view that ways compatible with the respect of human freedom and values must be found to prevent the tuberculous individual from infecting his fellow men. And the results already obtained suggest that great strides can be made toward the eradication of tuberculosis from well-policed communities merely by a program of detection of tuberculous persons and by educating them to a sense of social responsibility.

The tuberculin test and X-ray photography are the main tools used for the detection of tuberculosis. Two different types of information can be derived from large-scale testing with tuberculin. On the one hand, the conversion of an individual from the tuberculin-negative to the tuberculin-positive state provides convincing evidence that this individual has been recently infected and requires medical supervision, although it does not necessarily mean that he is suffering from active disease. On the other hand, the number of tuberculin reactors in any given population gives a quantitative idea of the prevalence of tuberculosis, which permits following the changes of incidence with time. For example, there are certain parts of the United States, particularly in the Middle West and Northwest, where tuberculosis has now become so rare that less than 10 per cent of the young adults are tuberculin-positive. By contrast, the figure is still of the order of 90 per cent in many large cities of the world where the disease constitutes a major health problem. Whereas the tuberculin test provides an index of infection, X-ray photography of the chest is the most convenient and most sensitive tool for recognizing the existence of tuberculous lesions before any symptom has made the patient aware of his disease.[8]

Analysis of familial, social or professional associations of newly discovered cases of tuberculosis often reveals the source from which the disease was contracted—more often than not, a person who is expectorating tubercle bacilli without even suspecting it. Thus, detection of tuberculosis in its very early phase is of extreme importance, not only because it facilitates the treatment of the patient, but also because it helps in locating the spreaders of infection and in taking measures to protect those with whom they associate.

Ideally, public health methods for the control of tuberculosis aim at the detection of all the carriers of bacilli in the community. But the difficulties and cost of the task are stupendous, and beyond the present-day facilities of most public health services. The inadequacy of the situation is made evident by the fact that some 30 per cent of the individuals who die of tuberculosis in the large American cities are not reported as tuberculous during life! Before dying, each one of them serves as a focus of infection during many months at least and often for several years.[9] But the difficulties of the problem should not breed discouragement or be an excuse for negligence. The example of several communities of ordinary economic circumstances shows how far public health measures can go toward the eradication of tuberculosis. In Minnesota, for example, there are now areas where no child of primary school age reacts to tuberculin. This has been achieved by the relentless prosecution of a program based merely on the early detection, segregation and education of infected persons. In the Bornholm Islands, also, whole communities have been made essentially free from tuberculous infection by similar policies. The fact that children are less likely to contract infection in sanatorium towns, and other communities where tuberculous patients congregate, than in places where awareness and understanding of tuberculosis are less acute, is further evidence of the effectiveness of sanitary practices fostered by education of the public.

Sanatoria play an important role in the complex system of public health measures. First devised, and still primarily used, as havens where patients are sent to recover their health, they also help in protecting society against the spread of infection by segregating and educating the spreaders of bacilli. Tuberculosis being regarded as a social disease, most antituberculosis services and sanatoria are operated with public funds. But in return society demands of the patient that he develop a sense of responsibility toward his fellow men, and society often takes coercive measures whenever that sense of responsibility fails. In North Carolina, the tuberculous individual judged by the local health department to be a menace to his family or community can be committed to a prison located on the grounds of the state sanatorium if he refuses to accept treatment in the regular wards, and his sentence may last for the duration of the active phase of the disease. In Iceland also the police have legal power to isolate individuals regarded as infectious, and physicians may seek this aid to force medical examination on unco-operative patients.[10] Generally, however, no law is needed to compel the patient with active tuberculosis to take advantage of the shelters that modern societies offer him. The two letters, TB, still evoke in most men the same vague terror that made of consumption one of the most dreaded words of the nineteenth century. Now that the fear has been personified and the tubercle bacillus is known to be the villain, measures designed to prevent its spread have acquired the compelling strength of common sense.

CHAPTER XIII

Healthy Living and Sanatoria

THE KNOWLEDGE and traditions concerning the management of the tuberculous patient are now codified in the formula of sanatorium life.[1] Although there have been throughout history many types of institutions especially created for the care of consumptives, they differed somewhat in concept from the modern sanatoria. Thus, the great temples of Greek and Roman civilization received patients who stayed for only a short time to receive health from the Gods sojourning in these pleasant and salubrious places; the Saint-Marcoul Hospital was founded in 1645 for the care and isolation of the scrofulous patients who had come to Rheims to be "touched" by the king; in London the Royal Chest Hospital was founded in 1814, the Brompton Hospital for Consumption in 1841, and the City of London Hospital for Diseases of the Chest in 1848; but these were all hospitals and not places devoted primarily to a healthy way of life.

The first documented example of an institution for open-air treatment of tuberculosis is the Royal Sea Bathing Infirmary for Scrofula, organized in 1791 by Lettsom, a fashionable Quaker physician of London.[2] He had been convinced of the medicinal value of the sea air by another English physician, Russell, who had noticed that fishermen did not suffer from scrofula. Russell also claimed that scrofulous children sent to him could be returned to their families after a season of sea bathing "the tumors of the neck cured, and their countenances healthy."

Lettsom was apparently in the habit of sending his wealthy

patients to the sea, and his philanthropic mind could not bear the thought that what was good for the rich was not available to the poor. One of the first, he had become aware of the misery and amount of disease in the fetid London tenements and had organized there a system of dispensaries. At Margate, a sea place chosen for the salubrity of its climate and for its easy access to the city, he established a hospital of thirty-six beds for the poor scrofulous persons that he examined in London. The hospital was so designed that patients could sleep on verandahs in the open air. In 1800 the hospital was enlarged to accommodate eighty-six beds and has continued to function and grow ever since.[3]

Despite its success, Lettsom's innovation did not spread and in particular did not affect the treatment of pulmonary tuberculosis. During the early nineteenth century, however, a few English physicians began to question the practice of keeping consumptive patients on a restricted diet in closed rooms. This change of attitude was a manifestation of the "sanitary awakening." The doctrine stated that pure air, pure water, pure food were essential to healthy living. But it was not easy to convince the official medical world that tuberculosis could be cured with such a simple formula. In fact, the Royal Academy of Medicine scornfully dismissed the possibility of treating the disease with fresh air in an official report stating that the view was five hundred years old and had long been discarded.

George Bodington is the best known and was the most bitterly attacked of those who taught that tuberculosis was curable by simple hygienic measures. His treatment was simple. According to him the most important remedial agent in the cure of consumption was . . .

> . . . the free use of a pure atmosphere . . . the air out of doors early in the morning either by riding or walking . . . with intervals of walking as much as the strength will allow of, gradually increasing the length of the walk until it can be maintained easily several hours a day.

To supplement this he recommended a bit of good wine to bring down the pulse of the patient, a good dinner to help him put on weight and an opium pill at night to make him sleep. He felt also that all this should be done under the direct guidance of the physician, preferably in a dwelling very close to his own.

> The abode of the patient should be in an airy house in the country; if on an eminence so much the better; the neighborhood should be high and dry; the soil a light loam, a sandy or gravelly bottom; the atmosphere is, in such situations, comparatively free from fog and dampness. Thus the equal temperature so much considered and said to be necessary should be that of the external air instead of that so commonly employed, the warmth of a closed room. . . .

In 1840 there appeared in the London *Lancet* a scornful account of the "very crude ideas and unsupported assertions" presented in Bodington's report. And for a few decades longer the medical profession continued to regard abundant food and fresh air as poisons for the tuberculous patient.

It is probable that despite official resistance, belief in the value of open air gained more and more adherents under the influence of the sanitary revolution. In 1853, for example, the Government of Lucca in Italy began sending scrofulous children to the sea baths at Viareggio.

The work of the German Hermann Brehmer marked the turning point in the treatment of tuberculosis throughout the world. Brehmer was born in Silesia in 1826, one day after Laënnec's death. Upon graduating from medical school, in 1853, he had devoted his doctoral dissertation to the theme that pulmonary tuberculosis is curable. His belief in the beneficial effects of life at high altitudes had been encouraged by his teacher J. L. Schönlein (who had introduced the word tuberculosis), and by the explorer Alexander von Humboldt who had assured him that the disease did not exist in mountainous countries.

In 1854 Brehmer established an institution for the treatment of tuberculosis at Görbersdorf in the mountains of Silesia. Opinion had now evolved sufficiently to welcome the new venture, and its success gave the needed impetus to the whole sanatorium movement. Yet it was a mistaken notion that had led Brehmer to search for the cure of tuberculosis in the mountains.[4] He had been impressed by the fact that, at autopsy, the heart of the consumptive was often found to be small and with weak muscular walls. Attributing this defect to poor circulation resulting from disease of pulmonary tissue, he concluded that it could be corrected by a healthy active physical life at high altitudes. Soon, however, he discovered by experience that vigorous exercise was harmful and he began to reduce the activity of his patients. Dettweiler, who had been a patient and a pupil of Brehmer, became even more impressed by the beneficial effects of rest. At Falkenstein in the Taurus Mountains he opened in 1876 a sanatorium of his own where he advised patients to rest for months on open-air balconies.

Within two decades the concept that tuberculosis could be healed by absolute rest in the open air was accepted all over Europe. The patient was moved from a stuffy, heated, tightly closed room to almost any place that afforded an atmosphere uncontaminated by civilization. The Swiss Alps were soon recognized as an ideal place in which to inhale "pure air," and the glowing reports of English physicians established their international reputation as health resorts.[5] Davos had been since 1841 a center for the treatment of scrofulous diseases, and it was there that Conan Doyle brought his tuberculous wife in the 1860's. John Symonds, Robert Louis Stevenson and other celebrities also came to Davos to take the cure and gave the Swiss sanatoria the literary glamour that received final sanction in Thomas Mann's *Magic Mountain.*

The change of attitude toward the treatment of tuberculosis is expressed with vigor in a guide book on Davos published in 1880.

> Consumption has always been too timorously, too leniently, too indulgently dealt with. Parents and doctors united to soothe the patient at Rome, and when the last stage was drawing nigh, sent him to end his sadly useless life, fittingly enough, in some romantic region. Davos demands qualities the very opposite of resigned sentimentalism in which too frequently the phthisical youth or maiden was encouraged. Here is no place for weak and despairing resignation; here you are not pusillanimously helped to die, but are required to enter into a hard struggle for life. . . .[6]

Not to be outdone, the lovers of the sea soon began to advertise the fact that the salt air had been known to perform miracles since antiquity, and hundreds of sanatoria sprang up along all the European shores. Little by little the sanatorium movement became more plebeian; fresh air was found to be good for the consumptive even if it was that of the ordinary countryside or of the large city suburb. Healthy living and rest in pleasant surroundings almost anywhere became the officially accepted treatment; and when George Bodington died in 1882, the *Lancet* published a laudatory obituary notice, the tone of which was in sharp contrast with the sneering account of his work published in the same columns forty-two years before.

In America it was the romantic life of Edward Livingston Trudeau which established the sanatorium movement and made of Saranac Lake and of the Adirondack region one of the greatest world centers for the treatment and study of tuberculosis. The details of Trudeau's life are widely known through his autobiography, and legend is already giving him a place beyond the confines of history. As had happened to Keats, it was probably while taking care of his consumptive brother that Trudeau contracted the disease that eventually assured him such a high place in the annals of medicine.

> I took entire care of him from the time he was taken ill in September until he died on December 23, 1865. We occupied the same room and sometimes the same bed.

> I bathed him and brought up his meals to him and, when he felt well enough to go down stairs, I carried him up and down on my back. . . . My sister and grandmother often sat with him in the daytime and allowed me to go out for exercise and change, but he soon became very dependent upon me and I had to be with him day and night. . . . I remember that, during the last week he lived, I had to drink green tea every night in order to keep myself awake but I held out to the end. . . . This was my first introduction to tuberculosis and to death.

Though slender, Trudeau was athletic, endowed with exceptional physical endurance, fond of hunting and of life in the wilderness. One night after walking from Central Park to the Battery in forty-seven minutes on a bet, he developed a vague illness. This was soon followed by the appearance of a cold abscess which had to be operated on several times before it healed. In those days the relation of such cold abscesses to tuberculosis was not understood, and little note was made of the incident. Two years later Trudeau suffered from other swellings of the lymph nodes in the neck, but like his first bout with the disease, this one also went unheeded. Failure to diagnose these first signs of tuberculosis are worth noting, all the more because Trudeau belonged to a medical family and was himself a recent graduate of the College of Physicians and Surgeons in New York. But according to his own account, his teacher had explained that tuberculosis "was a noncontagious, generally incurable and inherited disease, due to inherited constitutional peculiarities, perverted humours and various types of inflammation, and dwelt at length on the different pathological characteristics of tubercle, scrofula, caseation and pulmonary phthisis." Soon, however, Trudeau began to feel seriously ill and to suffer from attacks of fever that could not be relieved by quinine. When he finally sought medical attention, extensive tuberculous disease was found in the left lung.

As was still the fashion, he was advised to go South and try horseback riding. Failing to improve on this treatment, he returned to New York, taking exercise whenever he felt like it, but his health grew steadily worse and the outlook now seemed hopeless. Believing his end near, he decided to retire to the Adirondacks where he had spent some of the happiest days of his life in the past. It was not the thought that the climate would benefit him in any way that prompted his choice of the woods. The Adirondacks were then a rough, inaccessible region with a trying climate, but they were a paradise for hunters and fishermen. "If I had but a short time to live I yearned for surroundings that appealed to me and it seemed to meet a longing I had for rest and the peace of the great wilderness." And thus began his second experiment, of which he expected little except the undisturbed quiet of a remote place in which to linger until death should end the scene. Burning with fever, weighing "no more than a dried lamb-skin," he arrived at Paul Smith Inn on a beautiful June day. There he spent the summer resting, floating over the lakes, hunting and fishing from boats manned by devoted guides. Within a few months he had gained fifteen pounds, recovered his usual vigor, and was able to return to New York. Soon, however, the fever returned and early in June he set out once more for the Adirondacks, this time with his family. The miracle repeated itself. "On several occasions I have been taken to Paul Smith's from Saranac Lake in the Spring so ill that my life was despaired of; and yet little by little, while lying out under the great trees, looking out on the lake all day, my fever has stopped and my health slowly begun to return. . . . Again imperceptibly the fever began to fall, and strength — and with it the desire to live — to return."

In 1882 Trudeau read an account of the therapeutic results obtained by Brehmer in his sanatorium in Silesia. It inspired him to organize in the Adirondacks a similar institution, in the hope of allowing patients of moderate means to benefit by his own experience. With funds obtained from his wealthy friends, he began on a very small scale the Adirondack Cottage Sanatorium at Saranac Lake, now known the world over as the Trudeau Sanatorium. In 1882 Trudeau learned of the discovery of the tubercle bacillus by Koch. With an astonishing self-confidence, he arranged in his home a primitive laboratory and began to train himself in the new science of bacteriology. It seems that he was the first on the American Continent to cultivate a pure culture of the bacillus. From these pioneering efforts was born the Saranac Laboratory, still today a great center of tuberculosis research.

Trudeau wrote at the end of his life:

> Optimism is the one thing that is within the reach of us all, no matter how meager our intellectual equipment, how unpromising our outlook at the start, or how obscure and limited our careers may be. It was about my only asset when I built my first little sanitarium cottage on a remote hillside in an uninhabited and inaccessible region. Viewed from the pessimist's standpoint, that little cottage as an instrument of any importance in the warfare against tuberculosis must have appeared as a most absurd and monumental folly. Optimism made me indifferent to neglect and opposition and blind to obstacles of all kinds during the long years of struggle before the value of sanitarium treatment became generally recognized. It enabled me to undertake the culture of the tubercle bacillus and delve in the complex problems of infection and artificial immunization, though I had no knowledge whatever of bacteriology, no laboratory, no apparatus or books. It has steadily upheld my faith in the possibility of ultimately attaining to an immunizing treatment for tuberculosis, in spite of many discouragements and years of fruitless work.
>
> Optimism enabled me to assume for over a quarter of a century the financial support of my work, and though the little cottage grew to be a village, and the workroom in my house became a well-equipped laboratory, though their support each year required large and increasing sums, these have ever been forthcoming.

Progressive changes have been taking place during recent years in sanatorium life. As a reaction against the stuffy, overheated rooms of bygone days, patients were at first made to take the outdoor treatment whatever the weather. Wide-open windows and cure on outside balconies were the order, bleak and cold as the night or day might be. The art of wrapping oneself in blankets became an essential part of the cure, almost a ritual. Like any new drug, fresh air was taken with a vengeance. More conservative views now prevail.

Even for the consumptive the heroic days are over; life in the sanatorium is becoming softer. Concepts of rest and graded exercise are also evolving, presenting subtle problems of adjustment. How often the movies? How long the radio? How much eye and nervous tension dare one devote to TV? And what books are good to read for the sake of health — should the philosopher-patient relax with Kant, the mathematician with Einstein, the teen-ager with *True Love?* Or should the subjects of interest be reversed, and no one allowed to read or talk shop? [7]

In final analysis, the management of the consumptive in the sanatorium aims at a healthy, restful, peaceful life, the life that normal men should live if they were sensible. It is not a particular climate or a rigid formula of behavior that makes the sanatorium a haven for the tuberculous patient. It is an atmosphere of peace and repose, the mood that Shelley experienced in the "Euganean Hills":

> Soft sunshine and the sound
> Of old forests echoing round
> And the light and smell divine
> Of all the flowers that breathe and shine:
> We may live so happy there,
> That the spirits of the air,
> Envying us, may even entice
> To our healing paradise
> The polluting multitude.

Part Four

TUBERCULOSIS AND SOCIETY

CHAPTER XIV

The Evolution of Epidemics

TUBERCULOSIS has waxed and waned several times in the course of human history. In England, as we have seen, the mortality from pulmonary diseases seems to have been very high around 1650, then to have decreased slowly for many decades before climbing to a new peak before the middle of the nineteenth century. Death records from several countries of Western Europe and from the Eastern cities of North America reveal that a definite downward trend became manifest sometime after 1850. The decrease has continued ever since, at a remarkably constant rate, except for local and temporary disturbances in areas suffering from wars and revolutions. (Appendices A and B.)

It is customary to express death rates in terms of number of deaths per year per 100,000 population. Thus, the annual tuberculosis mortality rate for the combined populations of Boston, Philadelphia and New York was approximately 400 per 100,000 in 1830. In 1950 it was 26 per 100,000 for the population of the United States as a whole, and less than 10 in certain Midwestern and Western States. Although widespread, the downward trend did not begin exactly at the same time, and has not been proceeding at the same rate, in all the different countries of the Western world. General trends can be conveniently illustrated in the form of a few curves. (Appendices A and B.)

A peculiar fact emerges from the study of mortality curves; namely, that tuberculosis began to decrease long before any specific measures had been instituted against the disease — indeed, before there was any scientific basis on which to formulate antituberculosis campaigns. The germ theory was not accepted in medical circles until 1880, and the tubercle bacillus was seen for the first time in 1882; the treatment and segregation of patients in sanatoria did not gain momentum until 1900; vaccination is only now coming into use and is not practised at all in some of the places where the mortality has reached its lowest level; as to therapeutic measures — like lung collapse, thoracic surgery, and the use of streptomycin and PAS — they are of too recent date to have played any part in the phenomenon. Thus, it appears at first sight as if tuberculosis had been conquered by the human race without benefit of medical attention! In fact, so unexpected was the decrease in mortality that occurred during the second half of the nineteenth century that it remained unnoticed for several decades. When the concerted social and medical efforts to control tuberculosis began around 1900, the annual mortality caused by the disease in America and England had already fallen to 200 per 100,000, half the figure reached a few decades earlier. But even at this lower level tuberculosis remained the greatest killer of the human race, and it is not surprising, therefore, that many physicians and public health officers remained for a time unaware of the downward trend that had begun spontaneously.[1]

Because early mortality records are not accurate, statisticians usually select the mortality rates prevailing in 1900 as a base line for preparing tables and graphs illustrating the course of tuberculosis. This has led to the erroneous impression that the change in mortality began with the new century, and was initiated by the antituberculosis campaigns. It is true that the role played by these campaigns has been and remains immense, but it would be unscientific and unwise to ignore the natural forces that, independent of conscious policies, had begun to alter the balance between the tubercle bacillus and man long before the microbiological era.[2]

* * *

Tuberculosis is not the only infectious disease that exhibits an apparently spontaneous ebb and flow. Most epidemics first appear in the form of a few sporadic cases; this early phase is followed by one of great prevalence and severity; then new cases become progressively fewer and fewer, the disease often taking a benign character before disappearing almost completely for a time. "Epidemic diseases, like empires, rise, decline and fall." The duration of the epidemic cycle is fairly characteristic for each type of disease provided human intervention does not interfere with its natural course. There are on record, for example, many outbreaks of epidemic influenza recurring at intervals of approximately twenty years: but it is probable that the profound changes in the distribution of populations and in medical practices during the past few decades will blur considerably, or even eliminate completely, the regularity of this epidemic cycle.

In the light of these facts, some epidemiologists regard the present very low levels of tuberculosis mortality as corresponding to the end of a natural epidemic wave, and it has been prophesied that the mortality curve may rise again during the second half of the present century. This theory of epidemic waves, with a complete cycle of approximately two hundred years, is based on extremely thin evidence, depending as it does upon the interpretation of data of questionable accuracy.[3] But even granting that tuberculosis has evolved according to a long-range cycle in the past, this does not mean that an inescapable fate condemns mankind to be the victim of it in the future. Cycles are determined by natural causes, and some of these can be altered by human intervention.

In order to account for the rhythmic course of epidemics, it has been postulated that changes occur spontaneously either in the virulence of the causative agent, or in the susceptibility of the population that it attacks. Tests in experimental animals have so far failed to give any indication that the virulence of tubercle bacilli has significantly decreased during historical times, or at least since the bacteriological era. Moreover, today, as in the past, tuberculosis manifests itself with extreme violence and destructiveness when it attacks populations newly exposed to it, or any group of people compelled to live under conditions of physiological misery. It appears certain, therefore, that the same breed of tubercle bacilli that caused the great White Plague of the nineteenth century is still at large in the world today.

But if the bacillus has not changed, its human host certainly has. There is no doubt that the response of man to the damage caused by infection is profoundly affected by many different factors, and that some of these have varied in the Western world during the last century.

All accounts published by physicians and laymen in the past emphasize the tendency of tuberculosis to run in families. It is now realized that familial occurrence is, to a large extent, the result of a common source of infection in the household; but it is also probable that the manner in which the body responds to infection is conditioned by certain inborn traits that are hereditary, and that often bind several members of a family to a common destiny of disease.

The theory of familial susceptibility has received support from experiments with animals. Thus, the resistance of sheep belonging to a Scotch breed susceptible to tuberculosis has been increased by crossing them with a more resistant Pomeranian breed. By selective inbreeding it has been possible also to produce several families of guinea pigs and rabbits, each exhibiting a characteristic behavior toward infection. True enough, none of the selected animals was endowed with absolute resistance, since the disease could be produced in all of them by using a large infective dose. Yet the differences observed between the selected "resistant" and "susceptible" families were sufficiently great to have been of significance under natural conditions of exposure to infection.[4]

In human beings, hereditary disposition is readily recognized among identical twins, who usually exhibit identical behavior toward tuberculous disease, even after having been separated for many years and having spent their lives in very different environments; identity of genetic make-up results in a striking similarity of signs and symptoms. However, it is much more difficult to demonstrate the role of inherited susceptibility and resistance in the general population, partly because genetic traits are distributed in such a complex manner that they fail to appear as a clear pattern, partly because the influence of environmental factors on the course of tuberculosis is so great as to mask the manifestations of hereditary characteristics. Nevertheless, the statistical study of a large series of cases provides fairly convincing evidence of familial susceptibility to tuberculosis.[5]

It is probable that any human being can become tuberculous if he is exposed to heavy infection while in a state of physiological misery; but it is also true that the inbred characteristics may, under less drastic circumstances, spell the difference between health and disease, between life and death. This fact may play a large role in changing the susceptibility of the population as a whole. While hereditary resistance allows a certain percentage of individuals to go unscathed through destructive epidemics, most of the susceptible die young, often without leaving any progeny. Thus, familial susceptibility during epidemics is bound to express itself in a smaller number of descendants; in extreme cases, certain tuberculous families may become extinguished within a few generations. Only those endowed with some degree of resistance can survive wherever infection is almost universal.

Selective elimination of the most susceptible human families is not the only means by which a widespread epidemic increases the resistance of the population, for there is evidence that repeated exposure to infection confers on the survivors an acquired immunity which supplements their innate endowments. As will be recalled, a mild tuberculous infection producing an abortive disease or a disease with a very slow course can induce a state of immunity against an infective dose large enough to overcome a normal individual. That most human beings living in urban societies undergo such mild infections is indicated by the fact that they become allergic to tuberculin without ever showing any evidence of clinical disease. This widespread process of immunization through the agency of accidental contact infections may have been particularly effective in certain age groups in the past. Since tuberculosis is rarely severe in children between the ages of five and twelve, it seems not impossible that contact with tubercle bacilli during that age period provides some immune protection for later life. As the great majority of children were exposed to many sources of contagion up to a few decades ago, the occurrence of abortive infections among those lucky enough to survive may have led progressively to the development in urbanized areas of a partially immune population.

Whatever the validity of this argument, and it is difficult to support it by convincing evidence, the hypothetical immunity derived from childhood infection will become less common as time goes on. In several parts of the world, increasing numbers of children remain negative to tuberculin until late in their teens and, therefore, give no evidence of having experienced any contact with tubercle bacilli.[6] As the populations reaching adulthood will constitute more and more a virgin field for tuberculosis, there will be increasing chances to observe whether abortive infections contracted during childhood were really of much significance in establishing a state of relative immunity.

Although it is difficult to evaluate the role of selection and immunization in checking the spread of epidemics, there is no doubt that tuberculosis usually exhibits a very acute course in populations newly exposed to it. Some of the most dreadful manifestations of tuberculous susceptibility in populations compelled to change suddenly their ancestral ways of life are to be found among the Indians of the North American Continent.[7] The descriptions left by the Jesuit fathers who explored the Great Lakes region indicate that there were some cases of glandular and pulmonary tuberculosis among the natives with whom they came into contact. But the disease was then extremely rare among them, so rare that it was thought for a time to have been brought to the American continent by the European settlers. Similarly scrofula was practically nonexistent among the roaming Indians of Oregon.

The first well-documented outbreak of tuberculosis occurred among a group of some two thousand eight hundred Sioux made prisoners of war around 1880. No obvious evidence of tuberculosis had been found among them at the time that they were compelled to move into barracks in the prison camp; but soon deaths, due to the disease in its most acute form, began to occur. They increased rapidly from year to year, reaching in 1913 a level approximately ten times higher than that observed in Europe during the worst of the nineteenth-century epidemics. Even more destructive was the epidemic that ran riot among the Indians of the Qu'Appelle Valley Reservation in Western Canada. The tuberculosis mortality rate among them reached a fantastic figure corresponding to 9000 per 100,000 — the highest on record anywhere at any time. This was barely three decades after these Indians had to abandon their free way of life in the prairie. The Navaho Indians suffered a similar fate — despite the blessings of the sunny, warm and dry climate of Arizona. Among them also tuberculosis became, and has remained ever since, the greatest cause of disease and death after they lost the freedom of their favorite hunting grounds and were confined to the reservation.[8]

Scrofula and other forms of tuberculosis were extremely rare among the South Pacific Islanders before they came into contact with European immigrants, but within a few decades tuberculosis was the cause of 40 per cent of all deaths in New Caledonia and Hawaii. Similarly, epidemics of acute tuberculosis have been frequent among African Negroes. In the years 1803 and 1810, the British Government imported 4000 Negroes from Mozambique into Ceylon to constitute new regiments. By December, 1820, disease, tuberculosis in particular, had destroyed more than 90 per cent of them. Tuberculosis ran a fulminating course, without any tendency to healing, in the Senegalese troops and in the Capetown Boys brought to France during the First World War, with large numbers of them dying of the typical galloping consumption of bygone days.[9]

European people of Celtic origin appear to be particularly susceptible to tuberculosis. Young Irish adults working in England during the last war suffered severely from the disease, and the incidence of tuberculosis among Irish nurses at the Brompton Hospital for Chest Diseases in London, has always been so high that their applications for employment are not considered with favor. But it is not the fair complexion, red hair and blue eyes of the children of Eire that make them easier prey to the tubercle bacilli than are their English and Scottish cousins. It is, probably, the fact that in Ireland only recently did industrialization begin the process of racial selection and of immunization that had occurred in most other parts of Europe half a century before.

Against this background of extreme susceptibility to tuberculosis of ethnic groups newly exposed to it, there are many examples of the fact that populations which have been in contact with the disease for many generations in congested cities are more resistant than are those emerging from farming or nomadic life.[10] This is apparent among the several ethnic groups of Jews recently settled in Israel. The Ashkenazim and Sephardim came to the Jewish state from the cities of Central Europe and of the Mediterranean basin where tuberculosis has been endemic for many centuries, whereas the Yemenite Jews immigrated from an agricultural region where tuberculosis was almost unknown. In the latter group are commonly observed the rapidly progressive forms of the disease, such as caseous pneumonia and miliary tuberculosis, with a mortality much greater than that prevailing among the other Jewish groups.

In very broad terms, then, it appears that urban or industrial societies have tended in the past to breed populations endowed with a high natural resistance to tuberculosis. This theory would account for the fact that Ireland and Norway, which were among the last countries in the Western world to become industrialized, did not reach the peak in tuberculosis mortality until about 1900, several decades later than the rest of Europe. In Japan also, it is only very recently that the mortality has begun to recede. The tuberculosis epidemic is in its early phase in much of Latin America. The infection level is still rising in sparsely populated rural areas, but the endemic phase has begun in crowded urban districts. In Chile, for example, very recent surveys indicate that practically all persons over twenty years of age show evidence of having been infected. On the other hand the mortality in that country has been decreasing steadily from close to 500 per 100,000 of population in 1945 to approximately 300 in 1950, indicating that the relationship between tubercle bacillus and man is beginning to change. The history of tuberculosis in different human populations makes it plain that racial susceptibility or resistance is to a very large extent a consequence of social history.

Granted that the past history of a given population influences the response of its members to tuberculosis, it is also true that living conditions are of paramount importance in determining the severity of this response. Thus the tuberculosis mortality in the 1920's among the Jews living in the old and congested downtown Gouverneur District of New York City was 83 per 100,000, whereas it was only 52 in the newer and more open Bronx-Tremont District. Racially, the people were the same, but living conditions were much better in the new part of the city. At about the same period the tuberculosis mortality among the Irish of recent immigration was almost twice as high in the large

American cities, where they suffered from all the hardships of tenement life, as in their native country where most of them were rural dwellers. Although tuberculosis has certainly existed for countless generations in the large Chinese cities, it is there today a terrible scourge, causing a large percentage of nonpulmonary lesions and death at an early age in the poor classes. Their long history of contact with the disease fails to express itself in increased resistance, probably on account of their wretched economic status.

One of the most interesting examples of the effect of social and economic factors on the severity of tuberculosis is found among the Bantu populations in South Africa. The Bantus working in Johannesburg and other cities often exhibit an acute form of the disease and the tuberculosis mortality among them is one of the highest, if not the highest at the present time in the world. When severely sick, many of them return to their native villages (kraals) and certainly spread the infection among their kin before dying. Yet it appears that the tuberculosis mortality has remained extremely low among the Bantus who remain in the kraals, where they retain their ancestral way of life in a social structure based on family associations. If published statistics are correct, the Bantu is resistant to infection in his native social environment and highly susceptible to it under urban conditions in the same sunny South African climate.[11]

Wars usually bring into sharp relief the failure of hereditary resistance and of immunity when environmental conditions become too trying. Tuberculosis mortality increased suddenly and dramatically in Paris during the siege by the Prussian Army in 1871. Similarly, it increased everywhere in Europe within a very few months after the beginning of the two world wars — even in countries which did not take a direct part in the conflict and where food was never scarce. (Appendix C.) In many places forms of tuberculosis with a rapid course and without any tendency to healing became very common.[12] The tuberculosis mortality rates soared to levels even higher than those reached in the 1830's, and they soon reflected differences in the hardships suffered by the various groups of populations. During peacetime in Warsaw, the disease was less severe among the Jews than among the Gentiles; moreover, it had remained so during the First World War, although the mortality figures had increased sharply in both groups. Very soon after the beginning of the Second World War, however, the relation changed. From 71 per 100,000 in 1938, the tuberculosis death rate climbed to 205 in 1940 and 601 in 1942 among the Jews, whereas the respective figures were 186, 377 and 425 for the Gentiles. The resistance acquired during centuries of urban life in the crowded ghettos of Central Europe proved of little help to the persecuted Jew when his tragic load of ordeals became too heavy.

At the end of the Second World War tuberculosis had once more become the great plague of Continental Europe. But the threat of a lasting epidemic vanished as soon as living conditions improved and men began to live again in relative security. Many of those who had been near tuberculous death in the concentration camps succeeded in overcoming their disease when decent shelter, food and peace of mind were provided them; individual tragedies remained, but the over-all mortality rates resumed their downward trend. Thus, the course of tuberculosis during and after the war illustrates in a striking manner the powers at the disposal of the human body to master the disease when living conditions are favorable, but also the failure of native and immune resistance to protect against infection in the face of physiological and social misery.[13] (Appendix C.)

The tuberculosis death rates responded to the onset and to the cessation of the two world wars so rapidly as to make it doubtful that changes in exposure to the bacilli, in availability of food, or in working conditions could be the only factors involved in modifying the resistance of society to the disease. It seems that the severity of tuberculosis immediately reflects the complex of disturbances brought about in the community as a whole by most forms of social upheavals, be they abrupt changes in ancestral habits, rapid industrialization, or wars.

Obviously, the equilibrium between man and the tubercle bacillus is very precarious. If war can so rapidly upset it, other unforeseen events might also cause recurrences of the tuberculosis epidemic in the Western world. It would be of great help in social planning to know more precisely the circumstances which have suddenly decreased the resistance of European communities to tuberculous infection on several occasions during the recent past.

CHAPTER XV

Tuberculosis and Industrial Civilization

EACH AND EVERY VICE, large or small – in fact almost any form of unconventional behavior – was regarded as a cause of consumption during the nineteenth century. According to their personal prejudices, reformers and physicians traced the disease to immoderate love of food, spirits, or social life; to newfangled fashions, venery or lack of exercise; to excessive use of tobacco or a passion for dancing. The *Boston Medical and Surgical Journal* published a note in 1851 on the "Diary of a Tobacco Smoker and Chewer," said to be the veritable diary of the Reverend Solomon Spittle. The physician who performed the post-mortem examination had no doubt that the Reverend's death was due to "phthisis, caused by inordinate use of tobacco." When waltzing became the rage in the early 1800's, the new dance was regarded by many as the "ally of consumption and death." And a few decades later, the polka gained the name of "Polka Morbus" for being performed with a vigor considered dangerous.[1]

Discussing tuberculosis and heredity, Straham wrote in 1892, "This diathesis appears to be built up with equal certainty by impure air, drunkenness, and want among the poor, and by dissipation and enervating luxuries among the rich. From either set of causes it is capable of rapid development, and it is transmitted to the offspring with very great certainty. By injudicious marriages and persistent ignoring of the laws of health the necessarily fatal type is soon reached."[2]

Since tuberculosis was then almost exclusively an urban disease, there was ground for the universal belief that susceptibility to it was increased by the artificialities of city life.[3] In the United States in particular, it was easy to see the distemper advancing as the frontier life receded. "Phthisis . . . is scarcely known by those citizens of the United States who live in the first stage of civilized life and who have lately obtained the title of the first settlers," wrote Benjamin Rush in 1789. "It is less common in country places than in cities and increases in both." Tuberculosis was almost unknown among the early Ohio settlers. According to S. P. Hildreth:

> The invigorating effects of constant exercise, exposures to all kinds of weather, a simple, but nourishing diet, and the enlivening faculties of the mind kept in continual play, forbade the approach of this scourge of indolence, and the refinements of modern fashions. Very few cases of it occurred until after the year 1808 – and these did not average more than one death a year in a population of two thousand. Since the years 1815 and 1816 consumption has been gradually increasing, and at this time (in 1830) the average annual amount of deaths is about two in a thousand inhabitants.

Identical views were held by F. H. Davis in 1848.

> In the early settlements of this country, New England and the N. E. States were as free from consumption as are now the much vaunted far-western States and Territories. It was immediately consequent upon the change from an agricultural to a manufacturing population that the rapid increase in the death-rate from consumption is apparent in these States. Fifteen or twenty years ago Indiana, Illinois and the Lake region were the favorite resorts for consumptive patients. . . . Now we have a constantly increasing proportion of cases originating in this same region, not evidently from any change that has taken place in the climatic conditions, but from the change in the occupation and hygienic surroundings of the people.

In 1857, H. Gibbons pointed out that the disease had become established in California as soon as the population had increased in the coastal cities.

> A few years ago it was supposed that the climate of California was almost proof against Pulmonary disease. In 1850, if an individual happened to cough in church, all eyes were turned on him with curiosity and amazement. The native population, it was said, were entirely exempt from disorders of the lungs. But time has dispelled the delusions, and Pulmonary Consumption and the kindred affections, have become the great enemy of human life, as in the Atlantic States.

Only during recent decades has it become apparent that the spread of tuberculosis during the nineteenth century was the outcome of the social tragedies that followed in the wake of the industrial revolution, rather than the consequence of city life *per se*. The need for labor in the new factories brought about a huge and sudden shift of population from rural to industrial areas, an extraordinary migration of people which gave to Verhaeren's *Cités Tentaculaires* and to Goldsmith's *The Deserted Village* their dramatic atmosphere. In the mushrooming cities, the migrants found the most dreadful working and living conditions. Long hours of exhausting toil were exacted of them in the suffocating atmosphere of coal mines, in the dark factories and the damp offices. Malnutrition prevailed in the shabby, filthy and crowded tenements, and the bleakness of life was relieved only by gin and vice.

One of the most tragic aspects of early industrialization was the growth of child labor, particularly in the textile mills. As appears from an account published in 1795, the situation was already very bad in England during the late eighteenth century.

> Children of very tender age are employed; many of them collected from the workhouses in London and Westminster and transported in crowds, as apprentices to masters resi-

> dent many hundreds of miles distant, where they serve unknown, unprotected and forgotten by those to whose care nature or the laws had consigned them. These children are usually too long confined to work in close rooms, often during the whole night; the air they breathe from the oil employed in the machinery . . . is injurious; little regard is paid to their cleanliness and frequent changes from a warm and dense to a cold and thin atmosphere are predisposing causes to sickness and disability and particularly to the epidemic fever which so generally is to be met in these factories.

The working conditions for children were still as bad in 1838.

> The profits of manufacturers were enormous; but this only whetted the appetite that it should have satisfied, and therefore the manufacturers had recourse to an expedient that seemed to secure to them those profits without any possibility of limit; they began the practice of what is termed night-working, that is, having tired one set of hands, by working them throughout the day, they had another set ready to go on working throughout the night; the day-set getting to beds that the night-set had just quitted, and in their turn again, the night-set getting into the beds that the day-set quitted in the morning. It is a common tradition in Lancashire, that the beds never get cold.

Many of the mills were "dirty; low-roofed; ill-ventilated; ill-drained; no contrivance for carrying off dust and other effluvia; machinery boxed in; passages so narrow that they can hardly be defined; some of the flats so low that it is scarcely possible to stand upright in the centre of the rooms."

Although these descriptions probably represent the darkest aspects of child labor, its abuses were sufficiently general to prompt several inquiries. In 1843 the Children's Employment Commission on Trades and Manufactures published a report quoting examples of children working at the age of five, and stating that general regular employment began between seven and eight. It described the victims as . . .

> . . . stunted in growth, their aspect being pale, delicate and sickly, and they present altogether the appearance of a race which had suffered general physical deterioration. . . . The diseases most prevalent amongst them . . . are disordered states of the nutritive organs, curvature and distortion of the spine, deformity of the limbs, and disease of the lungs, ending in atrophy and consumption.

But, despite the report, child labor persisted uncontrolled for some twenty years longer.

Working conditions were equally bad everywhere in Europe and North America during the first half-century of industrialization. In the mills of Massachusetts and Connecticut, young women originating from rural areas worked all day long in an atmosphere which was "stifling and almost intolerable to unaccustomed lungs." After the day's work they retired to dormitories scarcely better ventilated than the mills. Four to six girls, and sometimes eight, slept in a room of moderate dimensions. The story is told of a manager who, attributing the morning "languor" of the operatives to a full stomach after breakfast, solved the problem by forbidding them to eat before work, and "succeeded in getting three thousand yards more of cloth a week for the same wagebill."

Within a few decades, millions of individuals raised on farms and in small towns were thus uprooted, and exposed suddenly to the debilitating effect of inhumane employment. In the United States, many of them were Irish emigrants who constituted an almost virgin field for tuberculosis. Friedrich Engels described, in *The Condition of the Working Man in England,* the "pale, lank, narrow-chested, hollow-eyed ghosts," riddled with scrofula and rickets, which haunted the factories of Manchester and other manufacturing towns. Living in slums and fed on bread, porridge and potatoes with very rarely some cheese and even more rarely a small bit of bacon, they typified the proletariat bred by the early phase of the Industrial Revolution all over the world.

The hardships caused by industrialization were not limited to poor lodging, inadequate food and physical exertion. Because man does not live by bread alone, standards of living cannot be defined merely in terms of crude economics. One of the worst evils of the Industrial Revolution was certainly to rob millions of human beings of the social and cultural values and of the emotional satisfactions which had made their lives bearable in the past. The most destitute villager in his native land had learned to adorn the dullness and drudgery of existence with bright ribbons and jolly tunes, and with the pageantry of his church. But when he was uprooted into the anonymous gloom of the industrial cities, it was only with the help of rum that he could escape from squalor and despair. Several generations would be needed for his descendants to reach the state of relative harmony that man can achieve with almost any environment.

Most of the new recruits to industrial labor had known poverty in their former rural surroundings, but their life there had been relatively free from stresses and physiological hardships. More important, they had achieved some sort of physiological and psychological adaptation to their humble social status. When they moved into industrial areas in search of prosperity, adventure and comfort, they found instead exploitation and other forms of poverty. And, while under stress, before having adjusted themselves to their new ordeals, they came into contact with city dwellers among whom tuberculosis had long been prevalent. Intense crowding in workshops and in unsanitary living quarters provided all that was required for the rapid spread of infection, while physiological misery favored the development of destructive disease. It is probably this constellation of circumstances which brought about the great epidemic of tuberculosis of the nineteenth century.

The association of tuberculosis with rapid industrialization can be observed again in several parts of the world at the present time. Large-scale migrations from rural areas to urban districts, disruption of ancestral habits and low standards of living—all these earmarks of the Industrial Revolution are now found in much of Latin America and of Asia. Concomitantly, tuberculosis is manifesting itself with the fulminating course that was so frequent in Europe and the United States in the 1830's, and the annual death rates are reaching 200 to 500 per 100,000 in the newly industrialized areas. (Appendix B.)

Long and strenuous working days, malnutrition, life amidst fumes, smoke and dust, seem sufficient reasons to explain the ravages of tuberculosis in the proletariat of the nineteenth century, but other causes must be found to account for the prevalence at the same time of fatal tuberculosis in the members of the more favored classes.

The mortuary registers for 1838 and 1839 in England reveal that the proportion of "consumptive cases" in "gentlemen, tradesmen and laborers" was 16, 28 and 30 per cent respectively. Thus, although tuberculosis affected the poor most severely, it was also a terrifying scourge in the well-to-do. The ever-recurring allusions to phthisis, chest disease, consumption, hectic fever, decline, through the diaries and other documents of the nineteenth century, bear witness to the fact that tuberculosis was ubiquitous, affecting young society women as well as their chambermaids and governesses; writers or musicians as well as unskilled laborers; physicians as well as their patients. It was the cause of tragedy, not only in the ghastly suburbs of industrial cities, but also in the small quiet towns, in the comfortable residential districts, and in the fashionable avenues of London, Paris, Rome, and New York. Exhausting physical labor was not demanded of the bourgeois and aristocratic classes; leisure and relaxation was their privilege; they were not displaced from their normal environment; their customs were not disturbed. But, at all levels of society, there were certain aspects of life that must have been directly and indirectly the cause of much infectious illness and of tuberculosis in particular.

In her *Life of Charlotte Brontë,* Mrs. Gaskell tells of the Brontë children being lectured, when they pleaded for more to eat, on the sin of caring for carnal things and of pampering greedy appetites.[4] Life in a girls' school was described as follows in the medical journal, the *Lancet,* of 1839:

> The girls rose at six and did preparation until eight, when they breakfasted on porridge, bread and tea. At 8:30 preparation was resumed until school began at nine, lessons continuing without a break until one. For half an hour they were free to leave the classrooms, but were not allowed to go out of doors. Dinner, consisting of boiled or roast meat, or boiled fish, and potatoes, with perhaps a suet or rice pudding to follow, occupied half an hour, and was followed by another three hours of school. Tea and bread were served at five; at six, if it were fine, the girls took an hour's walk, otherwise they stayed indoors and read.

The picture presented by Charles Dickens in *Oliver Twist* shows that half-starvation of growing children was a common practice of the time.

> The bowls never wanted washing. The boys polished them with their spoons till they shone again; and when they had performed this operation (which never took very long, the spoons being nearly as large as the bowls), they would sit staring at the copper, with such eager eyes, as if they could have devoured the very bricks of which it was composed; employing themselves meanwhile, in sucking their fingers most assiduously, with the view of catching up any stray splashes of gruel that might have been cast thereon.

The lack of elementary sanitation was beyond our most ghastly imaginings. Up to recent times, a group of children gathered in a closed room around a consumptive elder was regarded as a picture of poetical charm. Promiscuous spitting long remained as readily accepted as in the days when Samuel Pepys wrote in his diary, "I was sitting behind in a dark place, a lady spit backward upon me by a mistake, not seeing me, but after seeing her to be a very pretty lady, I was not troubled at it at all." The description of young schoolgirls drinking from a common cup appears as a matter of course in Charlotte Brontë's novels. These scenes betray an atmosphere of infection. Projected into the future, they take on the livid pallor of tuberculosis, and forecast young lives paralyzed or destroyed by disease.

The fact that tuberculosis was usually diagnosed only in its terminal phases also contributed much to its spread throughout the population, irrespective of social status. One often reads of the galloping consumption, so rare now under normal circumstances, but so frequent a diagnosis in the nineteenth century. The case of Keats dying within one year after becoming sick, with both lungs completely destroyed, is often quoted to illustrate the virulence of his disease. But wherever information is available, it takes little ingenuity to recognize that the tuberculous process had been going on for several years before diagnosis was made. Moreover, consumptive patients continued to live a life of normal activity almost to the end, not only spoiling any chance of arresting their own disease, but seeding the germs of it all around them. Galloping consumption was probably more the result of medical ignorance than of high susceptibility to infection.

The intensity of contagion must have been enormous. Keats, Poe, Thoreau and Trudeau nursing their dying brothers at home in small, closed rooms, without any precautionary measures; the Brontë children exposed for years to the chronic "bronchitis" of their father; the consumptive Virginia Poe giving singing parties only interrupted by profuse hemorrhages — these are typical examples of a behavior that was then commonplace. One reads of fashionable women in the last stages of consumption compelled by weakness to keep to their sick chambers through the day, but dressing at night to participate in social life and dying upright in the midst of festivities. In one of her letters, Thoreau's sister mentions a certain Ann K. Ford who had come to live as a boarder in their house in 1846. Ann was obviously consumptive, coughed incessantly, and suffered two serious hemorrhages in January, 1847. Yet she was cheerful, apparently unconscious of the seriousness of her situation, off visiting whenever she felt strong enough, enjoying in airtight rooms by hot stoves the company of her friends during the cold days of the New England winter. She died the following summer at the age of eighteen, having certainly contaminated many of her Concord neighbors and thus forged other links in the chain of contagion that was strangling New England.

In many places this lack of any awareness of the process of infection continued until the twentieth century. As late as 1899, Osler reported seeing in South Baltimore a lad, one of five children, who had been ill with tuberculosis for months. The room was stuffy and hot, both windows shut. Some expectoration was visible on the floor. "He had high fever, loss of appetite and was being fed on panopeptone and beef extracts. The room had a good exposure and I suggested to the young man to have the bed moved to the window, to be well covered up, and to rest in the sunshine during part of every day. The reply was that it would kill him and I could see by the mother's looks that she was of the same opinion. The doctor, too, I am afraid, regarded me as a fanatic."

It is probably this ubiquity of contagion that accounts for the prevalence of tuberculosis in the favored social groups during the Industrial Revolution. Physiological misery and crowding permitted the explosive spread of the disease among the labor classes, and from this huge focus the infection spread through society by means of countless unavoidable contacts. Interestingly enough this had been recognized as early as 1796 in the report of a commission appointed by the Manchester Board of Health.

"Children and others who work in the large cotton factories are peculiarly disposed to be affected by the contagion of fever, and when such infection is received, it is rapidly propagated, not only amongst those who are crowded together in the same departments, but in the families and neighborhoods to which they belong." However, the warning went unheeded. The passion for financial gains made acquisitive men blind to the fact that they were part of the same social body as the unfortunates who operated their machines. Tuberculosis was, in effect, the social disease of the nineteenth century, perhaps the first penalty that capitalistic society had to pay for the ruthless exploitation of labor.

CHAPTER XVI

Tuberculosis and Social Technology

THE SUFFERINGS and loss of human values caused by the industrial revolution were unnoticed at first by most of those who enjoyed the fruits of the new prosperity. But soon, the horrors of the manufacturing cities began to prey on the social conscience, and protests arose in every land.[1] These came not only from the victims, but also from representatives of the more favored classes. In England the Unitarian minister and medical man Southwood Smith and a few other physicians pointed out the iniquity and the dangers of the sordid conditions under which the masses of the people lived. Robert Owen proved by organizing model factories that humane standards of work in industry were not incompatible with financial success.

In 1837, the famous engineer Chadwick pressed for the appointment of a sanitary commission. The work of this commission led to the publication in 1842 of the *Parliamentary Report on the Sanitary Conditions of the Labouring Population of Great Britain.* In 1848 the Earl of Shaftesbury championed the establishment of the "General Board of Health" and fought for fair labor laws. Novelists, among them Charles Dickens, helped to arouse public conscience by portraying in graphic terms the evils of the time; Disraeli publicized child slavery in his novel *Sybil* and Charles Kingsley the sweated labor of tuberculous tailors in *Alton Locke.*

By 1850, reformers had come into action everywhere, attacking the social problems by political action, or devoting their efforts to improving the physical environment in which men had to live and function. Thus began a campaign to eliminate filth and squalor from society, to bring pure water, pure food and healthy living to the multitudes. Spitting in public places was taught to be a manifestation of bad taste, unguarded sneezing an antisocial act. Access to fresh air and sunshine became a natural right, good health almost a duty. It was this sanitary awakening, first championed by public-minded citizens, that paved the way for many of the advances in public health usually credited to the bacteriological doctrine.

The campaign for social reform gained momentum at the same time as the sanitary movement, the humanitarians joining with the labor organizations to demand a greater share of the new wealth for labor. Conditions improved in the factories and the working day was shortened. Wages increased and permitted better food in greater variety. Meat, dairy products, fruit and vegetables began to supplement the starchy diet which had been so long the main source of calories for the working man, and also the cause of deficiency diseases. More dwellings were built, even though dreary ones, and crowding decreased. It is worth noting that this movement was not built on a scientific doctrine. It sprang from humanitarian ideals and did not wait for the formulation of the germ theory of disease to preach that illness was, in large measure, the penalty of bad living and social injustice.[2]

Consumption was rarely mentioned in the programs of the reformers. Although the disease was ubiquitous and the greatest killer of the white race, its ravages were less obvious and less likely to produce hysteria than those of infections occurring as explosive outbreaks and causing rapid death. Epidemics of cholera and of yellow fever were short-lived and limited in space, but they exerted a terrifying impact on society because of their suddenness and destructive power; it was easy to single them out as well-defined events and to focus attention on them. Many of the regulations on which the present policies of sanitary control are based date from the cholera outbreak in Hamburg in 1892, and it was the threat of a new outbreak that led the municipal authorities of New York to establish a laboratory devoted to public health.

Tuberculosis, by contrast, appeared to be so constantly and universally present that there was a tendency to regard it as an act of God, affecting both the rich and the poor and against which little action was possible. Moreover, the disease was relatively slow in its course and did not produce repulsive lesions or symptoms. Pallor, emaciation, weakness, and even cough were actually considered fascinating in early Victorian days. "It is too bad," writes a modern historian, "that humans did not wear their lungs inside out as do certain species of amphibians, for in such a case the concern aroused might have demanded some sort of protection." [3]

This laissez-faire attitude was completely discredited by Koch's discovery. Bacteriological science showed that tubercle bacilli could be traced in their passage from man to man, and that they could be destroyed in transit. There, at last, was a target at which to shoot. By 1900, furthermore, it had become obvious that tuberculosis was most prevalent and most destructive in the poorest elements of the population, and that healthy living could mitigate its harmful effects. Reformers could attack the disease from two directions, by improving the individual life of man and by correcting social evils.

Pressure for some positive course of action was exerted everywhere as soon as practical knowledge became available. A "Society for the Establishment of Sanatoria for the Consumptive Poor" was formed in Austria in 1890, the "National League for the Campaign against Tuberculosis" in Denmark in 1891, and the "French League against Tuberculosis" the same year. Similar societies soon sprang up in Germany, Belgium, England, Portugal,

Italy and Canada. From the beginning, the antituberculosis campaigns carried immense social prestige. Royalty, chiefs of state, leaders of the political and social world personally presided over the meetings of the tuberculosis associations. The press gave wide publicity to the proceedings. The public was made aware of the magnitude of the ravages caused by the disease, and, fortunately, a partial solution to the problem could be presented in simple, comprehensible terms of wide social appeal.

The most important aspect of the movement was the eagerness with which laymen took part in it, often assuming leadership. Sociologists, philanthropists and businessmen did not behave as passive listeners when they came to sit with physicians in the committees organized to plan and instrument the antituberculosis campaign. In many places it was they, rather than the medical men, who initiated the new health movement, much as their forerunners had brought about the sanitary awakening in the 1840's. They were the voice of a farsighted citizenry who saw in tuberculosis a social disease that was not likely to be solved by a conventional medical approach.

Needless to say, individual efforts by physicians had not been lacking. A few dispensaries for treatment were in operation. Hermann Biggs of the New York City Department of Health had issued in 1889 an educational leaflet, *Rules to Be Observed for the Prevention of the Spread of Consumption,* which was a direct appeal to the people to participate in the fight against the disease. In 1892, Lawrence F. Flick had organized in Philadelphia the Pennsylvania Society for the Prevention of Tuberculosis.

The program of the new society, the first of its kind in the world, was so far-sighted that it provided a pattern eventually to be followed everywhere. It proposed to control the spread of tuberculosis

> (1) by promulgating the doctrine of the contagiousness of the disease; (2) by instructing the public in practical methods of avoidance and prevention; (3) by visiting the

> consumptive poor and supplying them with the necessary materials with which to protect themselves against the disease and instructing them in their use; (4) by furnishing the consumptive poor with hospital treatment; (5) by co-operating with boards of health in such measures as they may adopt for the prevention of the disease; (6) by advocating the enactment of appropriate laws for the prevention of the disease; (7) by such other methods as the Society may from time to time adopt.

According to Flick's own statement, "Great care was taken to exclude from the new Society all persons who were inimical to the contagious theory of tuberculosis." This was a wise move for, in 1892, many physicians still refused to believe in the contagiousness of the disease. As the program of the Pennsylvania Society envisaged the active participation of the general public, a systematic campaign of popular education was organized and laymen were invited to join with physicians in the antituberculosis work. To reach the populace a series of tracts was distributed on the streets and in drugstores, as well as through dispensaries.

Aside from these sporadic efforts, medical and public health bodies failed at first to take a vigorous, constructive attitude toward tuberculosis control. The first approach to an organized movement on a national scale in America came, not from clinicians in hospital or general practice, but from the Medico-Legal Society of the City of New York, a group composed principally of lawyers, scientists and physicians interested in social problems. In 1899 the Medico-Legal Society decided to organize an American Congress on Tuberculosis at which "the laws of the several states regarding the disease and its treatment" were to be considered. At a meeting held on February 22, 1900, the Congress of Tuberculosis went on record with the view that consumption was a communicable disease of social importance presenting the following questions to forensic medicine.

> 1. What legislation could be adopted by Congress or by the legislatures of American states that could possibly ar-

rest its ravages, prevent its spread and reduce the mortality among the people that had reached such alarming and amazing proportions? . . .

2. How could the masses of the people be educated up to be willing to vote for said legislations and to form a public opinion in America, among all classes of people, that could be relied upon to enforce such laws after they had been enacted?

This statement implied that the treatment and prevention of tuberculosis were matters that concerned the community as a whole, a principle that had been accepted in several European countries for almost ten years. It shifted the emphasis from treatment of the individual patient to the control of disease in society and involved a new relationship between the medical profession and the public. The whole community was expected to become familiar with certain technical problems of medicine and to take an active, constructive part in the campaign against disease instead of following passively the instructions of physicians. Commonplace as this point of view appears today, it was then a revolutionary departure in medical and social philosophy, one difficult to translate into practice. In fact, the concept was so new that it could hardly be defined in precise operating terms, let alone be enacted in the form of laws.

Ardent discussions enlivened by bitter conflicts of personalities continued for a few years in an attempt to reconcile the primary interest of practising physicians in the purely medical aspects of tuberculosis, with the insistence of public health officials and social workers on the educational and legislative approach to the problem. After much wrangling, a "National Association for the Study and Prevention of Tuberculosis" was organized in 1904. The word "Prevention" was pregnant with significance. It meant that the new society was to be an instrument of community action as well as of scientific study. In order to emphasize this fact, the secretary of the Committee on Organization elaborated on the program of the National Association in a public letter:

> I think I can safely speak for the committee in saying that one of the principal features of the contemplated work of the new society is to encourage social preventive measures. The title of the society as suggested will be the National Association for the Study and Prevention of Tuberculosis and its objects, as set forth in the by-laws, will embrace not only the scientific study of the disease of tuberculosis, but a study of all its relations to man, social and economic, and all measures for its prevention, eradication and cure.

This formula finally welded together the different phases of the antituberculosis movement and was adopted by the various national tuberculosis associations the world over. Public opinion was ready for the move, as is shown by the success of a pamphlet, *Tuberculosis as a Disease of the Masses and How to Combat It*, published in 1901 by A. S. Knopf of Philadelphia. "To combat consumption successfully," Knopf had written, "requires the combined action of a wise government, well-trained physicians, and an intelligent people." His pamphlet was translated into twenty-seven languages within a few years. Only the Bible had then enjoyed a wider distribution!

Public participation in the fight against tuberculosis soon took the concrete form of donations to finance the different phases of the work. The first appeal soliciting contributions from every purse, small or large, was made in Denmark, where the Christmas Stamp Sale was born in the mind of a postal clerk, Einar Holboell. In 1907 the idea was tested in the state of Delaware by Miss Emily Bissell, who thus raised 3000 dollars for a local tuberculosis project. Her success led the American Red Cross to experiment with the Christmas Seal on a national basis the following year, and the public response was immediately favorable.

In 1919 the Red Cross transferred the management of the Seal to the National Tuberculosis Association, which has had the responsibility of the program ever since. Christmas Seal Sales spread all over the civilized world, and their proceeds grew continuously from year to year. In the United States alone they amounted to more than $20,000,000 in 1950.

One of the most important activities of the antituberculosis associations has been to inform the public of the dangers of the disease. Judged by present standards, the publicity techniques used at the beginning appear somewhat crude.

> Some of us [writes a modern analyst of the movement] can still remember the empty-corner-beer-saloon tuberculosis exhibit, with its tuberculous and anthracotic lungs preserved in formaldehyde; with its jars of colored beads, each bead representing a soul victimized by tuberculosis; with its large painted skeletons depicting graphically the numbers annually dead of tuberculosis in the United States; with its flashing lights, each flash signaling the entrance of another soul into eternity *via* tuberculosis.[4]

As time went on, the program shifted from the fear motive to the promotion of understanding. The infectious nature of the disease, the properties of the tubercle bacillus, the factors that affect susceptibility and resistance to it, became the subject of lectures and of demonstrations that gave to children and adults alike some scientific basis for an intelligent attitude toward prevention and cure. This was the first systematic attempt at health education of the public.

The educational program is the basis of all other phases of the antituberculosis campaigns and has facilitated general acceptance of the various preventive and therapeutic measures described in earlier parts of this book. Health education has also had an indirect effect on social philosophy and practice, one that transcends in importance the control of tuberculosis. By teaching that disease is a community problem, not merely an individual experience, it has made of the preservation of health a responsibility of enlightened government. There is not one political party today that does not subscribe to this view.

Large departments, financed by Federal and state funds, are now applying on an ever-increasing scale the techniques of antituberculosis control slowly worked out during the past half-century. It is certain that this work will come to be recognized everywhere as a function of public bodies. But it seems doubtful that the unwieldy machinery of government would have been able to operate effectively during the early hesitating steps of the campaign. Although general agreement was soon achieved on broad principles, their application to particular circumstances presented many perplexing problems and it is fortunate that private agencies were then available to experiment with tentative policies first at the local, then at the national level. As we shall see, the social aspects of the tuberculosis problem are continuously changing. For this reason, the control techniques, and even the principles on which they are based, will have to be repeatedly altered to meet new circumstances and to incorporate new knowledge. It seems likely, therefore, that privately endowed and operated Health Associations still have a great role to play in spearheading the fight against disease along unorthodox approaches.

Fifty years have elapsed since the beginning of the concerted medical and social efforts to eradicate tuberculosis. Judged from the figures illustrating the continuous decrease in mortality, the results are overwhelming. But there are some epidemiologists who wonder whether the conscious antituberculosis measures really had much to do with the achievement. They point to the fact that countries which have engaged in large-scale campaigns and have the lowest mortality rates are also those enjoying the highest standard of living. According to their views, good food, decent housing, leisure, freedom from debilitating influences account for most, if not all, of the advances made against tuberculosis. In this light, detection of unsuspected cases by surveys, segregation of patients in sanatoria, and the various measures of prophylaxis and treatment would be luxuries in which a prosperous community can indulge, but which bear only an accidental relation to the decrease in mortality rates.

Other skeptics emphasize that tuberculosis mortality began to decrease in most places long before 1900 and that its downward rate has remained essentially constant, failing to reveal any obvious effect of the measures consciously introduced during the past decades. Furthermore, the decrease is occurring in several countries where the antituberculosis campaign is practically nonexistent, and the rate of decrease is not always the greater in those areas that have done the most to combat the disease. The discrepancy between results and expenditure of funds and efforts was recently emphasized in England by the Medical Officer for Cumberland County. Said he:

> Lancashire runs a model scheme. We do not pretend to do this. We have been prevented by economic depression. Why is it that Lancashire—which has a gross annual expenditure of 360,000 pounds compared with our 24,000 pounds on tuberculosis—has not, during thirty years, left us standing in this matter of death-rate statistics from tuberculosis? Why is it that with so many factors in the scales against us, we have, for a number of years, shown better, or more rapidly improving, figures than the average of the English counties? We are not in a position to claim any merit and I do not know the answer to these puzzling statistics and graphs.

Finally, it is becoming apparent that, simultaneously with the decrease in mortality of tuberculosis, there has taken place in much of the Western world a similar or in some cases an even greater fall in the mortality caused by other infections. This is true not only of intestinal diseases like typhoid fever or the diarrheas, which are transmitted chiefly by contaminated food and water, but also for measles, scarlet fever and the various forms of pneumonia, which, like tuberculosis, are primarily airborne. Particularly in the case of pneumonia has the fall in mortality rate followed a downward course which is almost indistinguishable from that of tuberculosis, and which began long before the introduction of serum therapy and the use of the sulfonamides or penicillin. Clearly, something has happened in the mode of living in our civilization which has rendered man more resistant to some of his ancient plagues. (Appendix A.)

While the skeptics are right in emphasizing the role played by natural forces in arresting the spread of tuberculosis, there are certain facts that throw a somewhat different light on the problem. First and foremost, it must be repeated that much of the program of education that has become such a cardinal part of the antituberculosis movement began long before the bacteriological era, with the great sanitarians of the early nineteenth century, and the reform of hospitals and nursing. It matters little whether crowding, promiscuous spitting, dark airless rooms, and other unsanitary aspects of life are condemned in the name of human decency, sanitation or the germ theory. The practical effects are the same in bringing about a way of life which minimizes the spread of certain infectious diseases and of tuberculosis in particular. It is true that the discovery of the tubercle bacillus gave a more rational basis to some sanitary practices and thus rendered them more effective. But, in reality, one can recognize a long unbroken continuity of public health work that antedates the microbiological era. The antituberculosis movement took up and carried further the torch first lighted more than a century ago.

In addition, the antituberculosis movement elevated the program of medical education of the public to a more sophisticated level. It conveyed the knowledge that disease can exist and can be detected long before there are any obvious symptoms. It taught that diagnosis in the earliest, asymptomatic phase of tuberculosis is of paramount importance, both for the individual patient, since it increases his chances of complete recovery, and for the community, since it helps in finding the source and breaking the chain of infection. The tuberculous patient has been indoctrinated in the belief that it is *his* responsibility to take measures to minimize the spread of bacilli, either by accepting segregation in a sanatorium or by learning to behave in such a manner that he does not contaminate his surroundings. It is true that most individuals with open tuberculosis long remain undetected and, unbeknownst to themselves, keep the disease going by infecting those with whom they come into contact.[5] Nevertheless, the experience of communities that have made an all-out effort to detect the spreaders of infection proves that the educational process can be highly effective.

Whereas the national death rate of tuberculosis for the United States was 22.2 per 100,000 population in 1950, it was 10 or less than 10 in Idaho, Iowa, Kansas, Nebraska, Utah, Wisconsin and Wyoming and had almost reached the vanishing point in certain parts of these states.[6] In the Western world, only those communities which have carried out systematic and sustained antituberculosis campaigns have come close to eradicating the disease. One of the most important achievements of the campaign has been the demonstration that, in the words of Hermann Biggs, "Public health is purchasable. Within natural limitations, any community can determine its own death rate."

Tuberculosis, it has been said, is a disease of incomplete civilization. Vague as this statement appears at first, it underlines the fact that the antituberculosis movement cannot be properly understood if seen only in its medical perspective, for the historical and social backgrounds loom large in the picture.[7] However desirable a goal, the complete elimination of tubercle bacilli is rendered impossible by economic and social factors. History leaves no doubt that, in their search for happiness or to escape from boredom, people will continue to crowd together and accept the risk of infection and disease. In most places, therefore, the immediate objective cannot be the eradication of tuberculosis, but merely how to minimize the burden that it places on man.

The problem of tuberculosis control is, of course, dominated by economic considerations. What is the cost of the disease to the community? How much can society afford to devote to medical and public health measures? Seen from a global point of view, for the world as a whole the situation is appalling. The estimates of annual death caused by tuberculosis vary from two to five millions, the number of persons totally or partially incapacitated by the disease must be ten times as great, and in most countries economic limitations prevent any effective methods of prevention or treatment. In India, for instance, there are one million deaths from tuberculosis every year. According to medical standards accepted in the Western world, this means that, at the very least, 500,000 beds and 15,000 doctors are required for antituberculosis work. In 1947, only 7000 beds and 120 doctors were available!

In the United States, five million persons have succumbed prematurely to the tubercle bacillus since 1900, but fortunately the prevalence of tuberculosis is now decreasing so fast that a number of epidemiologists have made so bold as to predict its eradication within a few decades. The mortality was only 34,000 in 1950. This rate, corresponding to 22 per 100,000 population, is indeed a vast improvement over the rates of 400–500 which prevailed a century ago. But satisfaction should not breed complacency. Although tuberculosis now ranks only seventh among causes of death in the United States, its importance is greatly magnified by the fact that it attacks large numbers of young adult persons. Among diseases it is still today the greatest killer for those between the ages of fifteen and thirty.

The real cost of tuberculosis is to be measured in terms of human values, not only of physical suffering, but even more of mental anguish, separation from loved ones, vanished hopes. This cannot be expressed in measurable units. It may be useful, however, to give a few figures illustrating the economic cost of the disease.[8] Inadequate as it is, the tuberculosis control program in the United States amounts to some 500 million dollars a year, making no allowance for hospital construction, depreciation of hospital buildings or training of specialized personnel. Pensions for veterans whose major disability is tuberculosis is of the order of 100 million dollars annually. The annual loss in wages, in production, in net future earnings by persons who die of tuberculosis or are incapacitated by it, runs certainly into many hundred million dollars. Tuberculosis is still the most costly disease!

Very disturbing also is the fact that the number of persons suffering from tuberculosis is not declining as fast as the death rate. While the number of deaths was 20 per cent smaller in 1950 than in 1947, the number of new cases reported increased in the same period. Obviously, we are more successful in saving people from tuberculous death than in preventing them from becoming tuberculous. "Is it not time that we raise our sights from the cemeteries and the premature graves to the living tuberculous who really need our attention and for whom we can still do something?" [9]

The problem of control presents itself in a very different manner, depending upon the stage of medico-social evolution of the community. Where the disease is extremely prevalent and awareness of its contagiousness is still lacking, no progress can be made until education has taught people to break the chain of infection in the household unit. In such places as certain Latin American and Asiatic countries, which are in the first phase of industrialization, the economic status of the destitute proletariat must be improved before adequate antituberculosis measures can be applied. Still another situation presents itself in the areas where the mortality is steadily decreasing but at an unequal rate in different social groups. For example, while the disease is now only a minor problem in certain parts of the United States, extremely high rates still prevail in the colored population; the death rate among whites is almost seven times higher among unskilled laborers than among professional persons, and twice as high among men as among women. Obviously, control work must be pointed to certain specialized parts of the population if further progress is to be made.[10] (Appendix E.)

Even if mortality rates continue to decrease, there will remain for many generations large numbers of tuberculous individuals who can be expected to live an almost normal span of life in equilibrium with their disease provided an adequate environment is given them. The fate of these chronic patients presents problems not answered by sanatoria, drugs, surgery, or collapse therapy, problems which will demand the formulation of new medico-social policies.

Several attempts have been made during recent decades to develop institutions where patients and former patients in all stages of recovery live under medical supervision while working at some gainful occupation. Examples of this program of rehabilitation in the United States are the Potts Memorial Hospital, which operates a printing department, and the Altro Workshop specializing in certain phases of tailoring. In Holland, there is attached to the sanatorium at Ber-en-Bosch a workshop where fine toys are manufactured for sale on the open market. By far the most comprehensive program is the Village Settlement scheme in Great Britain, which combines in a complete unit of operation the sanatorium, the workshops and the village. The industrial and farming activities presented at Papworth Village, Preston Hall, Wrenbury Hill and other places of this sort are manifold and pay wages that compare well with those prevailing in ordinary enterprises; moreover, the workers and their families receive the benefit of enlightened and ever-present medical services.[11]

This successful operation of the Village Settlement scheme in England demonstrates that there is room in the industrialized world for a compromise between the exacting requirements of competitive production and the restrictions that disease imposes on the tuberculous individual. It must be recognized, however, that the scheme has failed in countries other than England where it has been tried, and that its applicability is limited by many temperamental and economic factors. Rare are the semi-invalids who will welcome an environment where they can live in comfort but are set apart from the great common adventure in which their fellow men are engaged. Bold and imaginative experimentation is needed to develop social techniques permitting the tuberculous patient to function fully and safely, with normal social contacts, but without constituting a danger for the community.

Despite the effectiveness of antituberculosis campaigns in checking the spread of bacilli, the largest part of the population eventually becomes and remains infected, even in communities enjoying a highly developed public health program. It is probably safe to estimate that 1,000,000 individuals in the United States, and more than 100,000,000 in the world, harbor living virulent tubercle bacilli. In prosperous countries, the varied programs organized for the detection of active cases will bring to medical attention more and more patients in the early phase of their disease, and thus improve their chances of recovery. But disturbing problems are already becoming apparent. Recent surveys indicate that in New York and other large American cities, close to one thousand dollars must be expended to detect one new case of tuberculosis. This unit cost will probably increase as the prevalence of infection decreases and there is reason to fear that many communities will abandon too soon the search for active cases. In 1949, mass surveys by radioscopy in the

United States revealed 200,000 cases with lesions suggestive of tuberculosis. Yet only 14 million persons were tested — one tenth of the population! Complete medical examination of the suspicious but unproven cases would overtax the diagnostic facilities of the country. And the problem would be even more unmanageable in other parts of the world.

Furthermore, to what extent will society be willing, and able, to provide hospital or sanatorium treatment for all those who are infected and potentially dangerous? The cost would be staggering, perhaps exceeding a billion dollars yearly for the United States alone. And how many of the individuals found to have tuberculous infection, but otherwise feeling no unpleasant symptoms, will accept the idea of removing themselves from normal life for months or a year, merely as an insurance against the threat of disease? Only a very small percentage of tuberculous infections evolve into incapacitating illness, and there is at the present time no way of determining which of the infected individuals is threatened with progressive disease.

However useful in specialized cases, vaccination, antimicrobial drug therapy, or other therapeutic measures cannot possibly solve the *social* problem of tuberculosis. And yet it is certain that a solution can be found, for it must never be forgotten that tuberculosis is not an inevitable accompaniment of human life, as is shown by the fact that it has long been nonexistent in many primitive societies. While the passage from a rural to an urban and industrial type of civilization has been associated in the past with an increase in tuberculosis, it is now clear that industrialization or city life *per se* was not the determinant factor of the tragedy. As pointed out on several occasions, the incidence and mortality rates of tuberculosis have reached their lowest levels during recent years in some of the countries that are most thoroughly industrialized. In many areas, moreover, the disease is decreasing faster in large cities than in rural districts. Once the breeder of tuberculosis, the city may well turn out to be the final cleanser of it!

It is only through gross errors in social organization, and mismanagement of individual life, that tuberculosis could reach the catastrophic levels that prevailed in Europe and North America during the nineteenth century, and that still prevail in Asia and much of Latin America today.

In final analysis, the fight against tuberculosis can be carried along two independent approaches, by preventing the spread of the bacilli through procedures of public health, and by increasing the resistance of man through a proper way of life. Present scientific knowledge is almost sufficient to permit successful execution of the first part of the program, as shown by the fact that a few decades have sufficed to reduce infection to a very low level in communities that could afford to devote adequate resources to tuberculosis control. But, whereas the germ theory of disease gave a rational basis to the development of highly effective sanitary measures, no similar body of scientific doctrine has come to guide the antituberculosis movement in its efforts to render man more capable of dealing with the bacilli once contagion has taken place.

It is fortunate that the way of life affording greatest protection against tuberculosis is also well suited to fundamental happiness and health, for this has facilitated its adoption merely on the strength of common sense. Instructions against tuberculous disease need not read like coercive public health laws; they are identical with the rules of good physical living: cleanliness of body and habits, a room of one's own where sunlight and fresh air enter freely. Physical and mental rest can be regarded, not as therapeutic measures, but as necessities for normal human beings. Everyone agrees in principle that diets should be designed, not according to fads or outworn tradition, but in order to meet the unperverted demands of the body. Human activities are most satisfying when guided by physiological rhythms and by the moods of the seasons, rather than by the fashions of social coteries.

Useful as they are, all these wise recommendations add little to the teachings of the health crusaders in past centuries. Modern health pamphlets still read very much like the rules formulated by the monks of the Salerno School almost a thousand years ago:

> Let aire be cleere and light, and free from faults,
> That come of secret passages and vaults. . . .
>
> Use three Physicians still, first Doctor *Quiet*
> Next Doctor *Mery-man,* and Doctor *Dyet.*

Admittedly the medical techniques used in the management of the tuberculous patient, whether carried out in a city hospital or in a secluded country sanatorium, are of benefit to both patient and society. But it is probable that equally good therapeutic results could be obtained with more certainty, less time, and at lower cost of human and economic values, if knowledge were available of the factors that affect the course of tuberculosis. There is as yet no clear understanding of the specific mechanisms by which the body can ward off infection or progressive disease; there is no way of measuring either inborn resistance or acquired immunity; little more than lip service is paid to the need for investigating these problems. Yet it is likely that the point of diminishing returns will soon be reached in the beneficial effects to be expected from present practices. There is certainly more to physiological therapeutics than ill-defined "rest" and three square meals a day.

Elucidation of the mechanisms of tuberculous disease will long continue to require analysis by the methods of medical sciences. And the care of the stricken tuberculous patient calls upon all the resources of medical practice. But the complete control of tuberculosis in society goes beyond medicine in its limited sense. It is a problem in social technology.

Some fifty years ago men of vision and of good will, physicians and laymen, realized that tuberculosis could be conquered only by broadening the scope of conventional medical philosophy. Their efforts culminated in the educational program that enlisted the general public as an understanding and creative participant in the war against contagion. There is needed today a reawakening of the pioneering spirit that brought about first the sanitary revolution, and later the antituberculosis campaigns. Once more it becomes urgent to force upon social consciousness the realization that progress does not consist merely in doing more and more of what has proved profitable in the past.

A new process of education is needed to make the public, and those responsible for the administration of scientific programs – nay, the scientists themselves – become aware of the fact that research should not be limited to working out details of established principles, to gilding yesterday's lilies. The important advances are likely to come from the enterprising spirits who stray from the obvious paths and venture into unexplored land. It will take vision to foster the development of new points of view, within the ever-growing rigidity of our social framework, and it may prove difficult at times to integrate temperamental trail blazers in the rigid and cumbersome structure of large educational institutions and of governmental bureaus. But it also took boldness of spirit to establish in the 1900's the new philosophy that permitted physicians and the public to work together.

Needless to say, there is still much to be gained from exploiting the techniques of tuberculosis control that are the direct expressions of the germ theory of disease. But since the complete elimination of tubercle bacilli cannot be achieved during our lifetime or that of our children, it becomes imperative to investigate the human and environmental factors that determine resistance to infection. At the very dawn of the bacteriological era, Pasteur had stated with his vigorous and simple faith, "It is within the power of man to eradicate infections from the earth." Convinced as he was that germs can be harmful to man, he naturally pleaded for measures that would bring about their destruction or prevent their spread. But he also emphasized, over and over again, that physiological well-being and a healthy way of life could go far toward minimizing the harm caused by many infectious diseases. This is true of the infections caused by tubercle bacilli which, however widespread, are always less destructive in societies that live and function according to physiological common sense. The final step in the conquest of tuberculosis may well depend upon knowledge of the factors that prevent silent infection from manifesting itself in the form of overt disease.

It is entertaining and reassuring to discover that the laborious efforts made by medical science to eradicate tuberculosis have confirmed the value of certain ancient practices. Instinctively, or empirically, many primitive civilizations had developed the art of achieving fitness between human urges and the natural environment. We need to develop a new science of social engineering that will incorporate physiological principles in the complex fabric of industrial society. It will be the enviable task of the future to reconcile the glamour of modern life with the ancestral wisdom of the happy savage.[12]

APPENDICES

A. Long-range Trends of the Mortality Caused by Tuberculosis and Other Infectious Diseases

BECAUSE of difficulties of diagnosis, and for other reasons discussed in the text, early statements concerning deaths caused by tuberculosis are very inaccurate. Nevertheless, the outward signs of the *pulmonary* form of tuberculosis in its final stages are in most cases so obvious as to be readily identified.

Only the *deaths reported to have been caused by pulmonary tuberculosis* have been used in the preparation of Charts 1, 2 and 3, since other forms of tuberculosis were not diagnosed as such until a few decades ago.

Crude as they are, the values plotted in these charts clearly show that the number of deaths caused by tuberculosis began to decline in England and in the Eastern part of the United States sometime during the nineteenth century, even before the antituberculosis campaign gained full momentum. (The temporary increase in tuberculosis mortality which began around 1850 in the large cities of the United States is probably due to the sudden influx of Irish emigrants in that period.) The mortality caused by other infections of the lungs and of the intestines followed a parallel course, beginning to decrease before the introduction of specific therapeutic measures.

It is apparent that the decline in tuberculosis mortality is due in part to the same general forces which are progressively bringing several infectious diseases under control in the Western world.

The charts presented in Appendices A, B, C, D and E were drawn from data obtained from various sources. Most of these can be found in the writings of G. J. DROLET, J. B. McDOUGALL and A. R. RICH listed on pages 241 and 242.

Much useful information has also been derived from the book *The Burden of Disease in the United States,* by A. E. COHN and C. LINGG (1951).

We are indebted to MRS. SHIRLEY FERREBEE of the Tuberculosis Control Division of the United States Public Health Service for having made Charts 12 and 13 available to us.

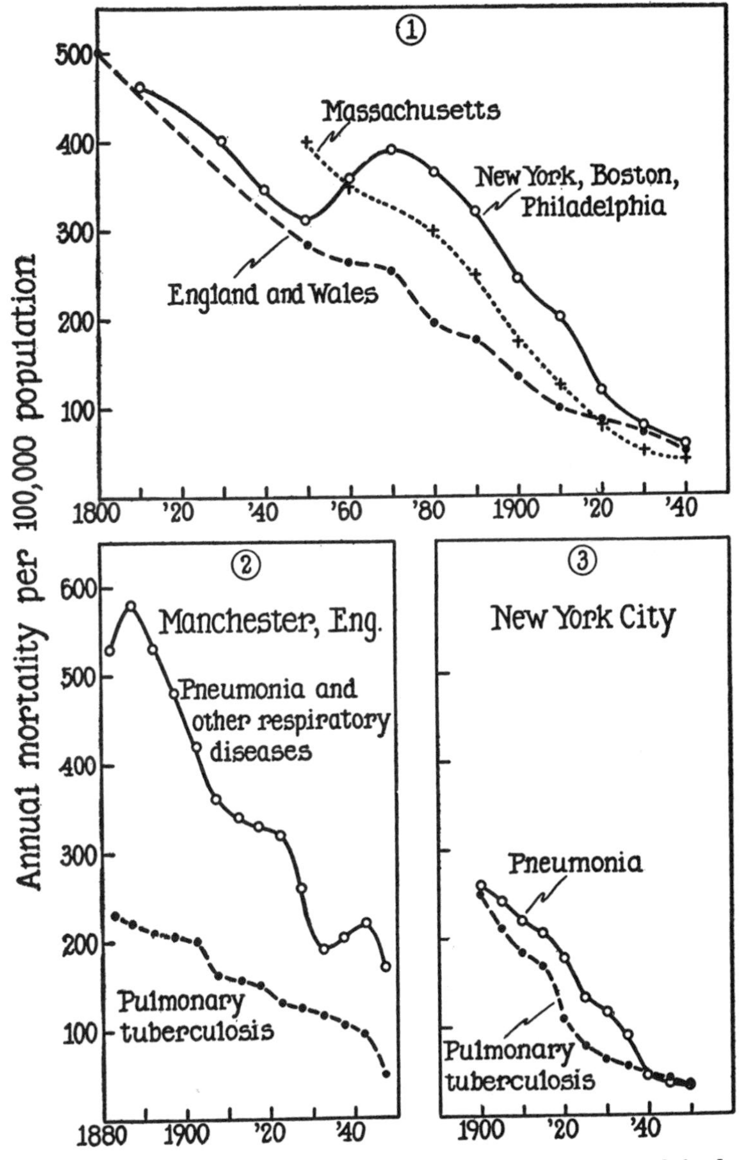

The figures at the bottom indicate the years, those at the left the number of deaths per year, per 100,000 population

B. Tuberculosis, Urbanization and Industrialization

THE VALUES plotted in Charts 4, 5, and 6 reveal a striking correlation between tuberculosis and the social structure. Death rates soared to their highest level shortly after the shift of national economies from the rural to the urban and industrial type. Countries which were the first to be industrialized also showed the first decline in tuberculosis mortality.

Although Denmark is usually regarded as an agricultural country, the fact that approximately half of its population lives in Copenhagen probably accounts for the fairly early peak of tuberculosis mortality in this country.

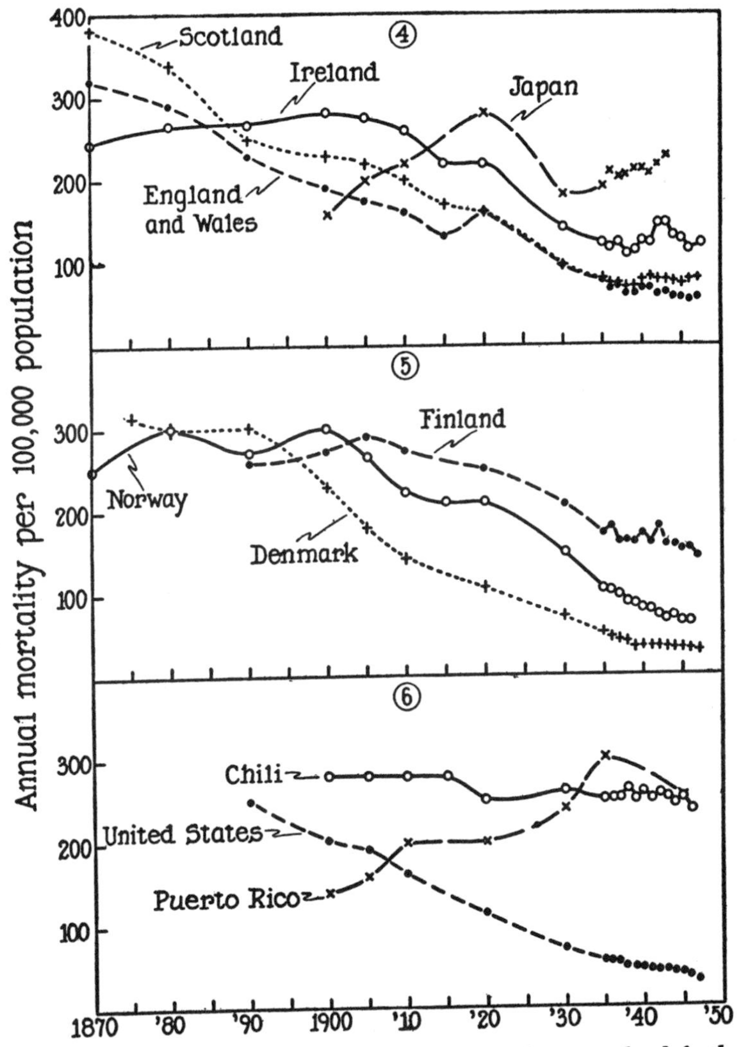

The figures at the bottom indicate the years, those at the left the number of deaths per year, per 100,000 population.

C. The Effect of War on Tuberculosis

Charts 7, 8 and 9 illustrate how rapidly the disturbances brought about by war are reflected in an increase in the number of tuberculosis deaths. By 1915, the tuberculosis death rate had increased in all countries at war — and even in some that had not yet taken part in the armed conflict. It is equally remarkable that the mortality curves began to resume their downward course in 1919, as soon as the war was over. In Prussia a new sharp increase in the number of deaths occurred in 1922 at the height of the inflation of the Germany currency.

As mentioned on page 141, the mortality in Denmark decreased after 1917, simultaneously with the interruption of the exportation of meat and dairy products by the submarine warfare.

In England, the increase in death rates during the Second World War was less striking than during the first. But although there was no large increase in tuberculosis mortality, it is obvious that the decline, which had been evident since the end of World War I in 1919, was suddenly interrupted in 1939, for a period of almost ten years.

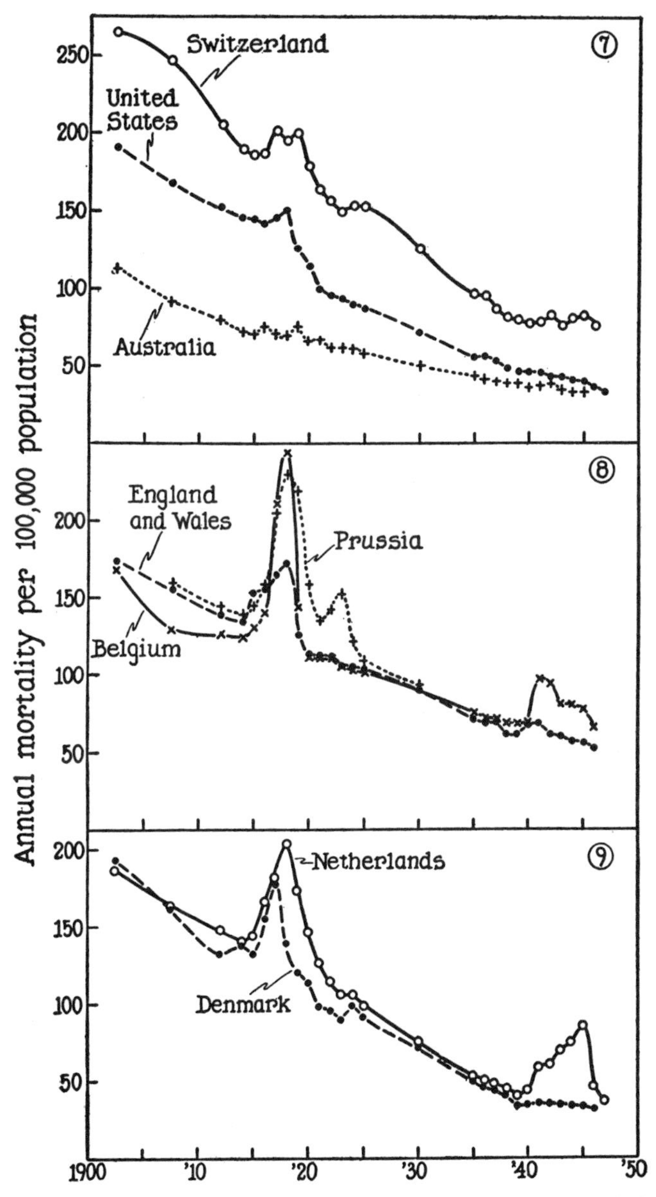

The figures at the bottom indicate the years, those at the left the number of deaths per year, per 100,000 population.

D. The Effect of Age on Susceptibility to Tuberculosis

CHILDREN between the ages of five and fifteen appear to be more resistant to tuberculosis than are adults or especially infants. This "golden age of resistance" was already clearly evident in 1900, at a time when infection was well-nigh universal. (Chart 10.)

The golden age of resistance is not peculiar to tuberculosis; it applies to many other infectious diseases as well, for example to pneumonia (and bronchitis) and to diarrhea (and other forms of enteritis). (Charts 10 and 11.)

The fact that children five to fifteen years old rarely *die* of tuberculosis does not mean that exposure to tubercle bacilli is without danger for them. Individuals infected at this age often develop progressive tuberculous disease later in life.

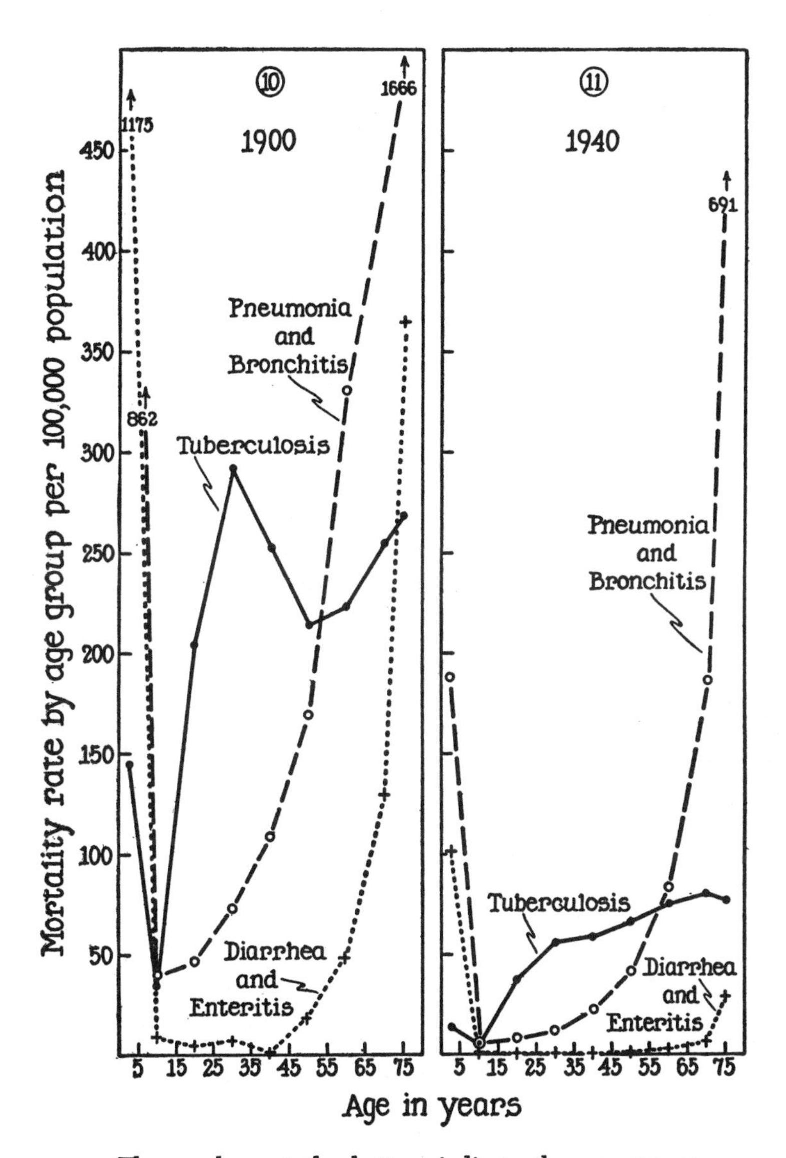

The numbers at the bottom indicate the age groups, those at the left the number of deaths per year per 100,000 population in each age group.

E. The Effect of Age, Sex and Race on Susceptibility to Tuberculosis

CHARTS 12 and 13 illustrate again the fact already shown in charts 10 and 11 that the lowest rates of tuberculosis mortality occur in children five to fifteen years of age; this is true for males and for females, among colored people as well as among white.

It is obvious that tuberculosis is still a problem of extreme gravity among the colored people in the United States, killing among them large numbers of young adults. Among white people, there has been during recent years a marked change in age distribution of the disease. More and more it is among older adults, particularly men, that tuberculosis finds its victims in the white race.

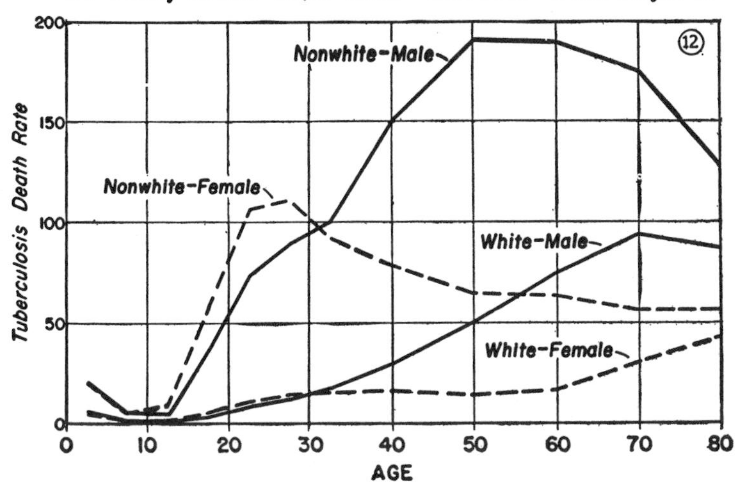

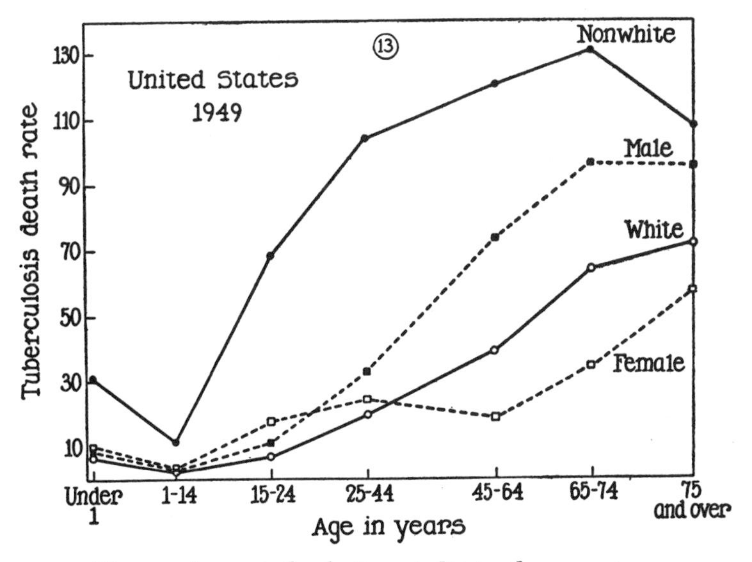

The numbers at the bottom indicate the age groups, those at the left the number of deaths per year per 100,000 population in each age group.

Bibliography and Notes

GENERAL REFERENCES

INFORMATION and detailed bibliographies concerning the early history of tuberculosis can be found in the following books and articles.

LAWRASON BROWN: *The Story of Clinical Pulmonary Tuberculosis.* The Williams & Wilkins Company, Baltimore, 1941

ARTURO CASTIGLIONI: *History of Tuberculosis.* Medical Life Press, New York, 1933

S. LYLE CUMMINS: *Tuberculosis in History.* Baillière, Tindall, Cox, London, 1949

LAWRENCE F. FLICK: *Development of Our Knowledge of Tuberculosis.* G. Dion & Cie., Paris, 1931

AUGUST HIRSCH: *Handbook of Geographical and Historical Pathology.* The New Sydenham Society, London, 1885, Vol. I and II

ANTOINE MERIUS PIERY ET JULIEN ROSHEM: *Histoire de la Tuberculose.* G. Dion & Cie., Paris, 1931

I. WALDENBURG: *Die Tuberkulose. Die Lungenschwindsucht und Skrofulose.* Hirschwald, Berlin, 1869

GERALD B. WEBB: *Tuberculosis.* Paul B. Hoeber, New York, 1936

Among recent texts in English presenting the modern knowledge concerning the medical, pathological, bacteriological and epidemiological aspects of tuberculosis, the following have been consulted most frequently during the preparation of the present volume:

GODIAS J. DROLET: *Epidemiology of Tuberculosis, in Clinical Tuberculosis.* Edited by Benjamin Goldberg. F. A. Davis Co., 1946

KAYNE, PAGEL AND O'SHAUGHNESSY: *Pulmonary Tuberculosis.* 2nd Ed. Oxford University Press, London, 1948

E. R. LONG: *History of Pathology.* The Williams & Wilkins Company, Baltimore, 1928

J. B. McDOUGALL: *Tuberculosis: a Global Study in Social Pathology.* E. & S. Livingstone Ltd., Edinburgh, 1950

ARNOLD R. RICH: *The Pathogenesis of Tuberculosis.* Charles C. Thomas, Springfield, Ill., 1944

NOTES

CHAPTER I

1. The descriptions of diseases of elephants given in the old Hindu literature indicate that tuberculosis was very frequent among these animals in India 2000 B.C. and earlier. See:

JOHN FRANCIS: *Bovine Tuberculosis.* Staples Press, London, 1947

2. In eighteenth-century London, families of good standing used to arrange through bribery that those relatives who died of syphilis be listed as victims of tuberculosis: See:

ERICH EBSTEIN: *Tuberkulose als Schicksal.* Ferdinand Enke Verlag, Stuttgart, 1932

3. The ebb and flow of tuberculosis in England during the past few centuries is discussed by:

J. BROWNLEE: *An Investigation into the Epidemiology of Phthisis in Great Britain and Ireland.* Medical Research Council, London, 1918

4. Much detailed information concerning the prevalence of scrofula in the world during the nineteenth century is presented by A. Hirsch in his *Handbook* (mentioned under General References).

5. Jenner believed that scrofula, "this formidable foe to health," had been rendered more devastating by the introduction of smallpox into Europe.

CHAPTER II

1. Information concerning John Keats (1795–1821) was derived from the following sources:

SHEILA BIRKENHEAD: *Against Oblivion. The Life of Joseph Severn.* The Macmillan Company, 1944

DOROTHY HEWLETT: *Adonais. A Life of John Keats.* The Bobbs-Merrill Company, 1938

WILLIAM HALE-WHITE: *Keats as Doctor and Patient.* Oxford University Press, 1938

AMY LOWELL: *John Keats.* Houghton Mifflin Company, Boston, 1925

JOHN MIDDLETON MURRY: *The Mystery of Keats.* Peter Nevill Ltd., London, 1950

2. Harvard men will be interested to learn that the name entered next to Keats's on the registration book at Guy's Hospital is that of the notorious John White Webster, who murdered a man and tried to dispose of the corpse chemically while professor of chemistry at the "Massachusetts Medical College."

CHAPTER III

1. ANDRE MERQUIOL: *La Côte d'Azur dans la Littérature Française.* Jacques Dervyl, Paris, 1949

2. For Nicolò Paganini (1784–1840) see:

F. J. FETIS: *Biographical Notice of Nicolò Paganini with an Analysis of His Compositions, and a Sketch of the History of the Violin.* Schott and Co., London, 1851

JEFFREY PULVER: *Paganini, the Romantic Virtuoso.* Herbert Joseph Ltd., London, 1936

3. See:

HEINRICH HEINE: *Florentine Nights*

4. For Rachel (1821–1858) see:

JAMES AGATE: *Rachel.* Gerald Howe Ltd., London, 1928

EDWARD ROBINS: *Twelve Great Actresses.* G. P. Putnam's Sons, New York, 1900

AUGUSTIN CABANES: *Poitrinaires et Grandes Amoureuses.* Les Laboratoires Cortial, Paris

5. For Marie Bashkirtsev (1860–1884) see:

MARIIA KONSTANTINOVA BASHKIRTSEVA: *The Journal of a Young Artist.* Translated by Mary J. Serrano. E. P. Dutton Co., New York, 1926

ALBERIC CAHUET: *Moussai, ou La Vie et la Mort de Marie Bashkirtseff.* Charpentier et Fasquelle, Paris, 1926

6. Among other Russians known to be tuberculous was Anton Chekhov. He was thirty-four when he appeared for the first time as a patient in the south of France in 1894. Later, he again came to spend the winter there, with a definite diagnosis of consumption. His health broken, he settled in Yalta, in vain seeking help from the mild Crimean weather. He died in July, 1904, in Badenweiler, a German health resort, whence he had come three weeks earlier to obtain medical assistance.

ANTON CHEKHOV (1860–1904): *The Personal Papers of Anton Chekhov*. Lear, New York, 1948

7. "The South" did not always mean some remote and exotic land. The novelist Charles Brockden Brown (1771–1810) was satisfied to travel no farther than from New York to Perth Amboy (New Jersey) to find a better climate to take the cure.

8. For Sidney Lanier (1842–1881) see:

VAN WYCK BROOKS: *The Times of Melville and Whitman*. E. P. Dutton Co., New York, 1947

SIDNEY LANIER: *Florida: Its Scenery, Climate, and History with an Account of Charleston, Savannah, Augusta, and Aiken; A Chapter for Consumption; Various Papers on Fruit-Culture; and a Complete Handbook and Guide*. J. P. Lippincott & Co., Philadelphia, 1876

EDWIN MIMS: *Sidney Lanier*. Houghton, Mifflin Company, New York, 1905

9. For Cecil Rhodes (1853–1902) see:

SARAH G. MILLIN: *Cecil Rhodes*. Harper & Brothers, New York, 1933

10. L. THAON: *Les Voyages en Mer et Les Poitrinaires*. Société des Sciences, Lettres et Arts de Nice, 1884

CHAPTER IV

1. Fracastorius, and many after him, had also reported the cases of several families whose members, down to the fifth or sixth generation, died of phthisis at approximately the same age (in their early thirties).

2. The following are a few among the many biographical studies on the Brontës:

PHYLLIS BENTLEY: *The Brontës*. A. Alan Swallow, Denver, 1948

LAURA L. HINKLEY: *The Brontës: Charlotte and Emily*. Hastings House, London, 1945

Ernest Raymond: *In the Steps of the Brontës.* Rich & Cowan, London, 1948

W. Bertram White: *The Miracle of Haworth.* E. P. Dutton, New York, 1939

Romer Wilson: *The Life and Private History of Emily Jane Brontë.* Albert and Charles Boni, New York, 1928

William Wright, Jr.: *The Brontës in Ireland.* D. Appleton and Co., 1893

3. Tuberculosis seems to have been common among the Brontës' acquaintances. Mary Taylor, who often slept with one of the girls at the parsonage, was thought for some years to be about to die of consumption. Ellen Nussey had fears of the same trouble and her sister spat blood. A young assistant rector looked pale and weak and died three years after his arrival.

4. For Ralph Waldo Emerson (1803–1882) see:

Haven Emerson: "Five Generations of Tuberculosis," in *Selected Papers,* W. K. Kellogg Foundation, New York, 1949

Regis Michaud: *Emerson, the Enraptured Yankee.* Harper & Brothers, New York, 1930

Ralph L. Rusk: *The Life of Ralph Waldo Emerson.* Charles Scribner's & Sons, New York, 1949.

5. For Henry David Thoreau (1817–1862) see:

Henry Seidel Canby: *Thoreau.* Houghton Mifflin Company, Boston, 1939

Joseph Wood Krutch: *Henry David Thoreau.* William Sloane Associates, New York, 1948

6. Without ever mentioning his own disease, Thoreau frequently refers to consumption in his *Journal.* In several places, he points out that the muskrats living in the banks of the Concord rivers never became consumptive despite exposure to severe cold and dampness. He gives this fact as evidence that muskrats are perfectly adapted to New England weather! On September 26, 1859, a few months before the beginning of his last illness, he makes the following entry: "The savage in man is never quite eradicated. I have just read of a family in Vermont who, several of its members having died of consumption, just burned the lungs, heart and liver of the last deceased, in order to prevent any more from having it."

See also quotes from Thoreau on pages 46 and 266.

CHAPTER V

1. Extensive lists of famous individuals who died of phthisis are presented by Ebstein, *op. cit.* (Chapter I, Note 2).

For general information concerning the literary mood of the nineteenth century the following books were consulted:

Albert C. Baugh: *A Literary History of England.* Appleton-Century-Crofts, 1948

A. Cabanes: *op. cit.* (Chapter III, Note 4)

Powell Spring: *Novalis, Pioneer of the Spirit.* The Orange Press, Inc., Winter Park, Fla., 1946

Paul Van Tieghem: *Le Romantisme dans la Littérature Européenne.* A. Michel, Paris, 1948

Van Wyck Brooks: *The World of Washington Irving.* Dutton, New York, 1944

C. H. C. Wright: *History of French Literature.* Oxford University Press, 1925

2. There were exceptions, of course, such as Keats's poem "To Autumn":

> Season of mists and mellow fruitfulness,
> Close bosom-friend of the maturing sun . . .

These lines illustrate the fact that, contrary to what is often believed, Keats's outlook remained more healthy than that of most of the romantic writers.

3. In fact, the opinion more generally held is, rather, that romanticism was one of the indirect causes of tuberculosis in the nineteenth century. Because it was fashionable among men to develop a passion for pale ladies apparently threatened with death, young women took to drinking lemon juice and vinegar as a means of killing their appetites. By extolling pallor, wrote a French commentator, Byron's poetry brought fortunes to grocers through increasing the sale of lemons! A "romantic dinner" was characterized by the affected indifference of the *convives* to the food. It seems not unlikely that many of those who regarded a consumptive appearance as the utmost in refinement and distinction eventually became victims of the real disease out of their efforts to play the part.

The desire to look emaciated was not entirely new in the history of fashion, for Montaigne had already written in the sixteenth century of women swallowing sand in order to ruin their stomachs and acquire a pale complexion. So repetitious are the tricks used by the sexes to attract each other!

It seems that eating heartily in public became good manners again sometime around 1840. "When I was young," wrote Théophile Gautier, "I could not have accepted as a lyrical poet anyone weighing more than ninety-nine pounds." But this attitude changed as the century advanced. Looking at all his successful contemporaries, Gautier came to the conclusion that "the man of genius must be fat." See:

LOUIS MAIGRON: *Le Romantisme et les Mœurs.* Librairie Ancienne Honoré Champion, Paris, 1910

LOUIS MAIGRON: *Le Romantisme et la Mode.* Librairie Ancienne Honoré Champion, Paris, 1911

4. Tsao (Hsueh-Chin) began writing his novel *Dream of the Red Chamber* probably in 1754; he died in 1763 having completed some 80 chapters and a general outline of the story. The novel was continued by others after his death. In *Armance, ou Quelques Scènes d'un Salon de Paris en 1827,* Stendhal pictures a woman who avoids mentioning the word "phthisis" for fear that it will hasten the course of her son's disease. Physicians attempt to reassure her by stating that the boy is merely suffering from the kind of "sadness which characterizes the young people of this era."

5. From "Consumption," by William Cullen Bryant.

6. *La Dame aux Camélias* was one of Sarah Bernhardt's favorite roles. The great actress also played the part of another consumptive character of historical and romantic fame, namely the Duke of Reichstadt (son of Napoleon I), in Edmond Rostand's *L'Aiglon.* The Duke died of tuberculosis in 1832 at the age of twenty-one.

7. It was probably this consumptive maid who served as model for the Goncourts' study of the degradation of a servant in their two novels *Renée Mauperin* and *Germinie Lacerteux.*

8. The Goncourts have provided many interesting details concerning the construction of their novel. They took two different women as models for "Madame Gervaisais" — their aunt for the psychological traits, and for physical appearance the wife of the celebrated chemist, Marcelin Berthelot. In the novel Madame Gervaisais dies as she enters the room to be received in audience by the Pope. In reality, their aunt died while dressing at home for this occasion. It is of interest that her child had shortly before died of meningitis.

The Goncourts explained the psychic effects of phthisis as due to "a slight intoxication, a loss of self-control, resulting from the semi-asphyxia caused by the accumulation of carbon dioxide gas that the lungs can no longer eliminate."

9. In his *Journal Intime* a consumptive Swiss philosopher, Henri-Frédéric Amiel, made the following entry on September 9, 1880: "It seems to me that with the decline of my physical strength, I am

becoming more purely spirit. Everything is becoming transparent to me. I see the types, the basis of living beings, the sense of things."

10. General information concerning the effect of disease on fashions and manners in the nineteenth century can be found in:

MAX VON BOEHN: *Modes and Manners of the Nineteenth Century as Represented in the Pictures and Engravings of the Time.* Transl. by M. Edwardes. E. P. Dutton & Co., New York, 1909–1927.

E. M. DELAFIELD: *Ladies and Gentlemen in Victorian Fiction.* Harper & Bros., New York, 1937

JAMES D. HART: *The Popular Book.* Oxford University Press, 1950

LOUIS MAIGRON: *Le Romantisme et la Mode.* Honoré Champion, Paris, 1911

LOUIS MAIGRON: *Le Romantisme et les Mœurs.* Honoré Champion, Paris, 1910

RUTH TURNER WILCOX: *The Mode in Costume.* Charles Scribner's Sons, New York, 1948

11. During the classical revival, it was fashionable for women to wear as little as possible. All clothing, including jewelry and accessories, was not to weigh more than eight ounces.

12. See:

HERVEY ALLEN: *Israfel: the Life and Times of Edgar Allan Poe.* Rinehart & Co., Inc., New York, 1949

13. See:

OSWALD DOUGHTY: *Dante Gabriel Rossetti – A Victorian Romantic.* Yale University Press, New Haven, 1949

VIOLET HUNT: *The Wife of Rossetti – Her Life and Death.* E. P. Dutton & Co., New York, 1932

14. Simonetta Vespucci, who inspired many of Botticelli's paintings, died of consumption at the age of twenty-three in 1475. Portraits of her were still being painted by Botticelli and his school seven years after her death. In a painting of her by Piero di Cosimo, a snake is shown stretching out his tongue toward her breast, a symbol of the disease that killed her.

15. There exists an enormous literature on the alleged relation between tuberculosis and genius. The following books provide interesting information on the subject and give extensive bibliographies:

GRAHAM BALFOUR: *The Life of Robert Louis Stevenson.* Charles Scribner's Sons, New York, 1915

Van Wyck Brooks: *John Addington Symonds. A Biographical Study*. Huebsch, Inc., New York, 1914

Erich Ebstein: *Tuberkulose als Schicksal*. Ferdinand Enke Verlag, Stuttgart, 1932

Jeannette Marks: *Genius and Disaster*. Adelphi Co., New York, 1926

Lewis J. Moorman: *Tuberculosis and Genius*. University of Chicago Press, 1940

Robert T. Morris: *Microbes and Men*. Doubleday, Page & Co., Garden City, New York, 1915

16. According to a recent author, *spes phthisica* may be merely the result of a suspension of critical faculties caused by anoxia of the prefrontal cells. See:

Maurice Porot: *La Psychologie des Tuberculeux*. Delachaux et Neufchâtel, Paris, 1950

17. Quoted from:

Arthur Maurice Fishberg: *Pulmonary Tuberculosis*. Lea & Febiger, New York, 1932

18. The literary view of the effect of tuberculosis on temperament and behavior is portrayed in the play *La Phalène*, by Henri Bataille. The life of the heroine of the play parallels that of Marie Bashkirtsev. Says the author, "I affirm that my heroine is drawn according to scientific truth. . . . She belongs to the intellectual tuberculosis type . . . great artists or great lovers, with their oscillations between strength and frustration, their enhanced nervous and creative life."

19. Many art critics have felt that the painter Watteau was influenced in the choice of his subjects by the fact that he suffered from tuberculosis. "L'embarquement pour Cythère," and other paintings, may have been the expression of his longing for a life from which illness excluded him.

20. See:

Lucy Poate Stebbins and Richard Poate Stebbins: *The Trollopes, the Chronicle of a Writing Family*. Columbia University Press, New York, 1945

21. Samuel Butler's *Erewhon* (1872) relates the trial of a consumptive whose disease is regarded as a crime. Butler took the judge's summing-up of the case from a contemporary newspaper report of the trial of a man found guilty of theft, with scarcely more alteration than the name of the offense. In Erewhon ill-health was punished as a crime, while those who murdered or stole were sympathetically

treated as ill persons. Criminals, according to Butler's view, were no more responsible for their actions than the Erewhonian son of consumptive parents was capable of avoiding his parents' disease. "Erewhon" illustrates the reaction against the romantic glorification of disease.

It seems that the sickly appearance began to go out of fashion in England before 1840, in certain social groups at least. When Chateaubriand visited London in 1822, "the man of fashion had to present the appearance of an unhappy and unhealthy man." In 1840 the French writer noted, "Today it is different. . . . His health must be perfect and his spirits always overflowing with five or six enjoyments."

In France, the change is apparent in the preface that Balzac wrote for his *La Peau de Chagrin*. "The public no longer wants to sympathize with the sick . . . the sad, the lepers, the langorous elegies." (See also T. Gautier's attitude, Chapter V, Note 3.)

22. See, for example:

Julien Green: *Adrienne Mesurat.* Librairie Plon., Paris, 1927
François Mauriac: *Le Baiser au Lépreux.* Editions Bernard Grasset, Paris, 1922

CHAPTER VI

1. It is worth noting that Flint and Welch soon afterward became leaders in the antituberculosis campaign based on the germ theory of disease. Welch was probably the first in the United States to demonstrate the tubercle bacillus to the students at Bellevue Hospital Medical College in New York.

2. This point of view appears with clarity in a letter written in 1783 by Beaumarchais to one of his friends suffering from phthisis. Beaumarchais expounds the doctrine of a physician who had been particularly successful in treating other cases of pulmonary consumption. "By concentrating on the parts of the body weak by nature, or weakened by accident, the acrid humors produce the ulcers of phthisis. As cough and spitting are only local manifestations of a more general disturbance, the ordinary remedies serve only as palliatives for the local disease, but do not reach its primary seat. . . . It is therefore necessary to redirect the course of the acrid humors in order to remove them from the weakened part of the body, and to throw them outside." This, according to the medical friend of Beaumarchais, could readily be done by a vigorous application of blisters over several parts of the body, the nearer to the location of the pulmonary lesion, the greater its gravity.

This letter from Beaumarchais was kindly brought to our attention by Professor Jacques Barzun. It is published in *Beaumarchais et son Temps,* by Louis de Léonie (Vol. II).

3. Although the adjectives "tubercular" and "tuberculous" are often used interchangeably in the lay and even in the medical literature, they convey essentially different concepts. "Tubercular" properly refers to lesions characterized by the presence of tubercles—whatever their causation. "Tuberculous" designates more specifically conditions produced by tubercle bacilli.

4. The word "apostheme" is often used in the old literature to designate a large deep-seated ulcer.

CHAPTER VII

1. See:

ALFRED ROUXEAU: *Laënnec Avant 1806 (1781–1805)*. Librairie J. B. Baillière et Fils, Paris, 1912

——: *Laënnec Après 1806 (1806–1826)*. Librairie J. B. Baillière et Fils, Paris, 1920

WILLIAM HALE-WHITE: *R. Théophile H. Laënnec.* Translation of selected passages from *De l'Auscultation Médiate,* with a biography. John Bale Sons & Danielsson Ltd., London, 1923

2. Resistance to the use of the stethoscope continued for several decades. Conan Doyle wrote of an English doctor who scornfully referred to the instrument as "a new-fangled French toy." Nevertheless, the doctor carried one in his hat "out of deference to the expectations of his patients, but he is very hard of hearing so that it makes little difference whether he uses it or not."

3. There was a young man in Boston town,
He bought him a Stethoscope nice and new,
All mounted and finished and polished down,
With an ivory cap and a stopper too.

It happened a spider within did crawl,
And spin him a web of ample size,
Wherein there chanced one day to fall
A couple of very imprudent flies. . . .

The doctors being very sore,
A Stethoscope they did devise
That had a rammer to clear the bore,
With a knob at the end to kill the flies.

Now use your ears, all you who can,
But don't forget to mind your eyes,
Or you may be cheated, like this young man,
By a couple of silly, abnormal flies.

4. A number of authors regard Laënnec's contribution to the field of tuberculosis as the turning-point in the study of the disease, and as having contributed more than any other to its understanding. See:

D. GUTHRIE: "Before and After Laënnec," in *Edinburgh Medical Journal* 53/12, 1946, 699–708

A detailed historical analysis of the concepts of the pathology of tuberculosis during the nineteenth century has been presented by:

ROSMARIE BISCHOFF: *Beitrag zur Geschichte der Kontroverse über die Natur des Tuberkels von Bayle bis Baumgarten.* Dietschi & Cie., AG., Olten, 1950

CHAPTER VIII

1. This state of affairs was still in existence on the Island of Cyprus a few years ago. The occurrence of multiple cases of tuberculosis in one family or community of families was still so common on the island in 1937 that physicians and laymen were convinced of the hereditary nature of the disease. In reality, the fact that the social and economic structure of Cyprus is based on very close family associations accounts in large part for the striking familial distribution of tuberculosis among the Cypriots.

2. It has been suggested recently that the gravity of phthisis in members of closed religious orders may be due in part to the unconscious wish of the victims to renounce earthly life. This mental attitude would render them less resistant to the effect of faulty hygiene and of inadequate nutrition. Thus, the young Carmelite nun, Sainte Thérèse de Lisieux, welcomed the onset of phthisis as a means to an early death and martyrdom.

3. In a collective investigation carried out in England in 1882, most physicians expressed disbelief in the contagiousness of phthisis, "The evidence of large institutions for the treatment of consumption such as the Brompton Hospital, directly negates any idea of consumption being a distinctly infective disease."

In the edition of his *Handbook*, published in 1885, A. Hirsch still doubted that "Koch's discovery of so-called tubercle bacilli in scrofulous glands" had anything to do with scrofula.

4. A recent discussion of the importance of Villemin's achievement will be found in S. Lyle Cummins's book (listed under General References) and in:

MAZYCK RAVENEL: "By-products of Tuberculosis Programs," in *Transactions*, 28th annual National Tuberculosis Association Convention, 1932

5. Surprisingly enough, there does not exist any full-size biography of Robert Koch. Valuable information concerning his life will be found in S. Lyle Cummins's book and in:

VICTOR ROBINSON: *Robert Koch.* Medical Life Press, New York, 1932

6. See:

H. R. M. LANDIS: "The Reception of Koch's Discovery in the United States," in *Ann. Med. Hist.*, 1932, 531

7. The precise history of the development of the Ziehl-Neelsen technique now commonly used for the staining of tubercle bacilli is somewhat unclear. In May, 1882, Paul Ehrlich published his paper showing that tubercle bacilli are not decolorized when treated by nitric acid after being stained with a mixture of gentian violet and anilin oil. Hence the expression "acid-fast" bacilli. Koch immediately accepted Ehrlich's method as superior to his own. Shortly after, Ziehl recommended that carbolic acid be used instead of anilin, and Neelsen suggested fuchsin and sulfuric acid to replace gentian violet and nitric acid. See:

WILLIAM BULLOCH: *The History of Bacteriology.* Oxford University Press, New York, 1938

Paul Ehrlich diagnosed that he had tuberculosis by finding tubercle bacilli in his sputum, stained by his own technique. Following this discovery, he spent a year resting in Egypt and came back to Germany with restored health.

8. The reasons which made Koch try to keep secret the nature of his "remedy" have never been made public. On several occasions Koch stated that the preparation of his material and the technique of its use required such skill that therapeutic accidents were likely to occur if the method were made available too soon to untrained practitioners.

It seems, however, that the policy of secrecy was dictated by the German Ministry of Health. There were rumors, according to the *Lancet* of 1890, pointing "to the intention of the German Government to retain, as it were, the monopoly of the remedy in its own hands . . . to become the proprietary of a vast patent-medicine factory."

9. See Character Sketch, "Dr. Koch," in *Review of Reviews* 2, July–December, 1890, 547.

10. Another early English medical visitor to Berlin was Sir Joseph Lister. He accompanied his tuberculous niece, who was to receive the tuberculin treatment from Koch himself.

11. The use of tuberculin in therapy has never been completely abandoned. Moreover, recent discoveries at the Radcliffe Infirmary, Oxford, England, indicate that the substance may find an important place in the treatment of tuberculous meningitis in conjunction with streptomycin.

CHAPTER IX

1. Because the exact time at which infection has taken place is usually unknown, it is difficult to determine the time sequence of the different phases of tuberculosis. In the few cases where precise information is available, the incubation period from infection to the first signs of disease (development of a positive tuberculin test, *hilum adenitis, erythema nodosum,* and other signs) has been found to range from two to seven weeks. The appearance of tuberculin allergy is accompanied by an infiltration around the primary tuberculous focus which renders the latter visible by X ray; there is some fever, rarely exceeding 102° F., and lasting three to ten days, with some anorexia and lassitude. The onset is usually so insidious that proper diagnosis is not made.

2. Approximately half of the individuals discovered to have active tuberculosis by routine surveys are entirely unaware of symptoms. Yet the disease is often in a moderately advanced or far advanced stage at the time of diagnosis.

Most of those who have symptoms fail to appreciate their significance and trace them to a variety of minor troubles — such as cigarette cough, sinus infections, nosebleed, bleeding gums, colds, grippe, overwork, poor food, bad digestion, unsanitary living or working quarters, and other ills.

3. The laryngoscope was devised in 1854 by García, a Spanish singing teacher residing in France. According to his own account, García had always had a great desire to visualize the larynx. While strolling in the Palais Royal in Paris, he "suddenly saw the two mirrors of the laryngoscope in their respective positions, as if actually present before the eyes."

4. In the case of tuberculosis, dependence of susceptibility on age is made even more striking if one analyzes the problem by determining the ratio of numbers of deaths to numbers infected in each group. Unfortunately, it is not a simple matter to recognize infection in the absence of overt signs of disease, as the test for tuberculin allergy, which is the only practical index of infection at the present time, gives results often difficult to interpret. Nevertheless, comparative surveys of mortality rates and of tuberculin allergy reveal differences which are sufficiently striking to appear significant. They show that, in 1945

(before the advent of drug therapy), the mortality rate was extremely high (of the order of 5 per cent) among infants below one year of age infected with tuberculosis. It fell rapidly to a very low level (0.02 per cent) until puberty, then increased again and oscillated around 0.07 per cent until death. This point is discussed by A. Rich, *op. cit.* (see General References).

5. The role of psychological factors (bereavement, disappointment in love, loss of fortune) in the causation of disease was accepted as a matter of course by physicians and laymen until the nineteenth century. The importance of these factors came to be neglected more and more during the period when medicine was dominated by the purely mechanistic outlook as a result of rapid advances in the sciences of pathology and microbiology. It is only during the past few decades that efforts have been made to develop techniques for recognizing, measuring, and analyzing the influence of psychic phenomena as causal agents of pathological disturbances.

6. When the great Spanish neuro-histologist, Santiago Ramón y Cajal, developed tuberculosis at the age of twenty-six, he was sent for treatment to a resort in the North of Spain. Despite his refusal to follow the rest cure, his health improved rapidly, a fact which he attributed to his taking up photography with passionate interest. See:

DOROTHY F. CANNON: *Explorer of the Human Brain: The Life of Santiago Ramón y Cajal (1852–1934)*. Henry Schuman, New York, 1949

7. In his *Morbus Anglicus,* published in 1672, Gideon Harvey presented a peculiar view of the pathology of tuberculosis, a typical example of substitution of words for factual understanding: "Melancholy calcined by the flame of choler must remain the sole cause of acrimony and corrosion. . . ."

8. The effects of the psychic state on tuberculosis, and of the disease on the mental reactions of the tuberculous patient, are discussed at length in MAURICE POROT, *op. cit.* (Chapter V, Note 16).

See also Chapter VIII, Note 2.

CHAPTER X

1. Several volumes would be needed to describe all the various remedies which have found favor at some time in the past for the treatment of tuberculosis. Two examples will suffice to illustrate the range of imagination of physicians at the end of the eighteenth century. Marat, who was a practising physician before becoming the fierce publicist of the French Revolution, had an "antipulmonic water," con-

taining chiefly calcium phosphate. It gained him the wealthiest and most elegant practice of Paris. Thomas Young was impressed by the beneficial effects of feeding daily to consumptive patients an extract prepared by boiling down a quarter of a pound of mutton suet in a pint of milk.

A review of some of the folk practices used in the treatment of tuberculosis is given by:

J. D. ROLLESTON: "The Folklore of Pulmonary Tuberculosis," in *Tubercle,* March, 1941, 55

Drinking the blood of a recently slaughtered animal is one of the practices which has gained acceptance in many countries. In fact, there is an authentic report of a crime committed in Andalusia to provide a tuberculous patient with fresh human blood. "A boy of eight years was seized one evening, gagged and put in a sack. He was then taken to the patient's room, undressed and then, without being moved by his cries and prayer, the quack plunged his knife into his left axilla. The patient then drank his blood while the boy was dying." This incident is reported by:

J. BERCHER: "Los Curanderos," in *La Presse Médicale,* April, 1939, 606

2. This practice apparently persisted through much of the nineteenth century. In *La Peau de Chagrin,* Balzac speaks of a Swiss consumptive who cured himself by breathing in, extremely slowly, the "thick air of a cowhouse."

3. There were many who held that the beneficial effects of sea voyages on phthisis were due to seasickness and could be obtained by swinging. Erasmus Darwin suggested that results as good as those of swinging could be obtained by provoking nausea through the rotary motions of a chair some thirty times a day.

4. In 1865, A. Sax, Jr., published a booklet entitled *The Gymnastic of the Lungs. Instrumental Music Considered from the Hygienic Point of View.* See:

LEON KOCHNITSKY: *Adolphe Sax and His Saxophone.* Belgian Government Information Center, New York, 1949

5. Asses' milk was already much in vogue in the eleventh century in the School of Salerno.

In Great Consumption learn'd Physicians thinke,
'Tis good a Goat or Camels milke to drinke
Cowes'-milke and Sheepes' doe well, but yet an Asses
Is best of all, and all the others passes.

In England, "The Family Oracle of Health" published a recipe for preparing an artificial asses' milk to be used in cases of consumption. "Bruise eighteen garden snails, with one ounce of heartshorn shaving, an ounce of eryngo root . . ." and so on.

CHAPTER XI

1. When ice cream was introduced shortly before 1880, it was found to have "the happiest effects in checking the irritation of the cough and abating the violence of the hectic."

2. See:

J. B. Orr and J. L. Gilks: "The Physique and Health of Two African Tribes," *Medical Research Council, Special Report,* Series No. 155, London, 1931

The relation of food supplies to tuberculosis in various European countries during the two world wars is discussed in McDougall's *Tuberculosis,* page 359.

3. At the present time, some of the highest tuberculosis mortality rates are observed among the Eskimos in the frozen North, the Bantu Negroes in dry sunny Africa, the Hindus in tropical humid India, the whites in the island of Cyprus or in Latin America. By contrast, very low mortality rates are observed among special groups of the same races living under these very same climates. Clearly, the role of climatic and racial factors is small in comparison with that played by economic and social conditions.

4. In the 1860's H. I. Bowditch published a number of epidemiological studies to support his view that residence upon a damp soil was a potent factor in the production of consumption, whereas residence upon a dry soil aided in the cure of the disease. See for example:

Henry I. Bowditch: *Consumption in New England and Elsewhere.* David Clapp & Son, Boston, 1868

5. Here should come a discussion of the importance of sound sleep for health in general, and for resistance to tuberculosis in particular. Unfortunately, while there is universal agreement on the beneficial effects of sleep, there is no knowledge concerning either its mechanism or its physiological role. The modern physician has little to add, beyond high-sounding words, to what Thomas Dekker wrote in 1609 in *The Gull's Hornbook:*

. . . sleep is that golden chair that ties health and our bodies together. Who complains of want, of wounds, of cares, of great men's oppressions, of captivity, while he sleepeth? Beggars in their beds take as much pleasure as kings. Can we therefore surfeit on this delicate ambrosia? Can we drink too much of that whereof to taste too little tumbles us into a churchyard, and to use it but indifferently throws us into Bedlam?

6. Locke himself suffered from tuberculosis throughout his life; his father and brother died of it. Sydenham advised him to go to bed early, speak as little as possible, eat and drink light, take up horseback riding and spend winters in the South of France.

7. See:

W. C. GREENHILL: *Anecdota Sydenhamiana.* London, 1845

8. "I always find," wrote John Addington Symonds, "that to organize a big book drills the holes in my lung. The other part of the business bores the body out, but does not destroy tissue."

9. The development of the various techniques of pulmonary collapse and of thoracic surgery is described in detail in Lawrason Brown's book.

Soon after Forlanini's papers, intrapleural pneumolysis by galvanocautery was devised to cut the pleural adhesions which, in many cases, prevent satisfactory collapse of the diseased areas. Extrapleural pneumothorax was advocated to separate completely the diseased lung from the chest wall. Thoracoplasty, the resection of ribs overlying a lesion, which had been practised on a limited scale since 1885, received a new impetus from the interest in artificial pneumothorax after the development of roentgenology had made it easier to control the operation.

Collapse of the lung can be brought about indirectly by therapeutic pneumoperitoneum which consists in instilling air into the abdominal cavity. Pneumoperitoneum causes the diaphragm to rise to a higher position in the chest and thereby reduces the space occupied by the lungs between the fixed apex at the top and the diaphragm below. The diaphragm is composed of a sheet of muscle enveloped in two membranes, the pleura on the chest side, the peritoneum on the abdominal side. As it offers much resistance to the stretching effect of the introduced air, collapse is often facilitated by crushing the phrenic nerve and thus paralyzing the muscle on the right or left side of the neck. In other words, phrenic paralysis in combination with pneumoperitoneum increases the extent of pulmonary relaxation or collapse on the more diseased side of the lungs.

While thoracoplasty brings about a permanent and complete deflation of the part of the lung over which it is performed, both pneumothorax and pneumoperitoneum possess in common the theoretical advantage that they are reversible procedures, since the lung tissue should be able to reexpand and function again after introduction of air is interrupted. Unfortunately, this hope is not always fulfilled and there often occur in the collapsed lung profound changes which destroy irreversibly its respiratory functions. In consequence, collapse procedures are now regarded as somewhat less advantageous and less safe than was assumed some two decades ago.

CHAPTER XII

1. Recent observations have established that the development of resistance to streptomycin by tubercle bacilli is markedly delayed when patients receive PAS at the same time as the former drug. Many studies are under way to determine the optimal indications for this combined form of therapy.

Several other drugs have been shown to exert a therapeutic effect in mice or guinea pigs, but none has yet proved as useful as streptomycin and PAS in human tuberculosis. At the time of writing, isonicotinic acid hydrazide, also known as Nydrazide or Rimifon, has been tested with encouraging results, on a limited scale.

2. Vaccines made of killed tubercle bacilli have recently been used on a fairly large scale in human beings in Jamaica and in Italy, with encouraging results.

3. See:

E. L. Trudeau: "Two Experiments in Artificial Immunity against Tuberculosis," *Trans. Nat. Ass. Study and Prev. Tub.*, 1905, 157

4. Several experienced clinicians have emphasized the fact that miliary and meningeal tuberculosis have all but completely disappeared from communities which have engaged in a systematic program of vaccination with BCG. It is true, on the other hand, that these diseases are also practically nonexistent in the white population of large cities such as New York and Philadelphia where vaccination has not been practised to any significant extent.

5. See:

John Francis: *op. cit.* (Chapter I, Note 1)

6. Human disease caused by bovine tubercle bacilli is extremely rare in the United States, but fairly common in England and Scotland, particularly in children under the age of fifteen. Bovine tuberculosis is somewhat less frequent in Wales. At least two factors may account for this difference: the much higher proportion of tuberculosis

in cattle in England than in Wales (21.3 per cent as against 5.4 per cent in 1949); and the practice of pasteurizing milk in the larger towns of South Wales.

In many countries where tuberculosis is still common in cattle, the incidence of infection caused by bovine bacilli in human beings is kept low by the practice of boiling milk before consuming it.

In 1847, the English journal, the *Lancet,* suggested that bad milk might be responsible for scrofula in man. It was then difficult in London to find a sample of milk which did not show some blood and pus on microscopic examination.

7. An idea of the prevalence of tuberculosis in cattle during the nineteenth century can be gained from the following incident. In 1890, Queen Victoria ordered that the dairy cows on the Home Farm at Windsor be tuberculin tested. Thirty-five of the forty cows were found to be tuberculin-positive, and tuberculous lesions were found in all of them! And yet "the premises on which these cows were kept were probably the best in the kingdom, and the general cleanliness left nothing to be desired." See:

J. FRANCIS: *op. cit.* (Chapter I, Note 1)

8. Despite the fact that over 500,000 chest X-ray examinations were made in New York City in 1947, this technique of screening detected only a small percentage of the total number of new cases of tuberculosis registered that year. Moreover, it was found that, contrary to hopes, the proportion of tuberculous individuals discovered in the early or minimal stage of their disease was smaller than in preceding years; more than 75 per cent were in the second or third stage when first detected! Clearly, a great deal remains to be done in our large cities toward the development of techniques for early detection of tuberculosis.

9. It is generally agreed that in most communities, there are at least ten active cases of tuberculosis for each death from the disease. In the United States, the registration of new cases corresponds only to three times the number of deaths, evidence of the fact that many active cases remain undetected. Moreover, in a large series of autopsies carried out in New York on persons dying suddenly of causes other than tuberculosis, it was found that almost 5 per cent had lesions (including cavities) showing active and often advanced tuberculous disease which had remained unsuspected.

10. Court action for the commitment of persons with infectious tuberculosis, who endanger the health of the public, was provided by the 1951 Minnesota legislature. Under the new law, the county board, on the health officer's report of a suspected tuberculosis case, may commit such a person by resolution. If the person refuses treat-

ment, court action is prescribed and appeal is provided, but commitment is not stayed unless ordered by the court.

If a patient willfully violates sanatorium regulations or leaves without consent, he may be charged with disorderly conduct and, upon conviction, may be confined in disciplinary quarters set up at the state sanatorium or other institution.

CHAPTER XIII

1. Although the word "sanitarium" is often used in place of "sanatorium," the two words differ in origin. "Sanitarium" comes from *sanitas* (health), "sanatorium" from *sanare* (to cure, to heal). The German physicians seem to have preferred the latter word, perhaps to express the view that cure in a sanatorium implies a positive therapeutic intervention, and not merely the beneficial effects of life in a healthy environment.

2. In addition to his fashionable practice in London, his medical work for the poor and his particular attention to the problem of scrofula, Lettsom had many other activities. He was one of the first to come out in favor of Jenner's vaccination, and he founded the Medical Society of London at the age of twenty-eight. But, despite all his important achievements, he is remembered chiefly because of the rhyme:

> When any sick to me apply,
> I physics, bleeds and sweats 'em.
> If after that they choose to die,
> Why Verily!
>
> I LETTSOM

See:

JAMES JOHNSTON ABRAHAM: *Lettsom, His Life, Times, Friends and Descendants*. William Heinemann, London, 1933

3. In his essay, "The Old Margate Hoy," Charles Lamb describes a poor lad on his way to the infirmary for sea-bathing at Margate. "His disease was a scrofula, which appeared to have eaten all over him. He expressed great hopes for a cure." The voyage from London took one or two days and nights.

4. See:

ADOLPHUS S. KNOPF: "The Centenary of Brehmer's Birth." *Am. Rev. Tub.* 14, 1926, 207

5. However, Jenner advised John Addington Symonds to spend his winters on the Nile, after passing a few weeks in the Alps as a preliminary tonic. When Symonds decided to stay in the mountains, Jenner wrote him, "If you like to leave your vile body to the Davos doctors, that is your affair; I have warned you."

6. In addition to these general views, the author presents many specific reasons to account for the beneficial effects of curing at Davos. Vague and unproved as they are, his theories are of interest in reflecting contemporary opinions concerning the causes and cures of tuberculosis.

"Dryness of air absorbs suppuration, the purity of atmosphere and its consequent freedom from germs, permits the internal wounds to heal and encourages cicatrisation; the rarity of air acts upon the respiratory organs as a species of gymnastic exercise . . ." The author emphasized the importance of walks in pine forests with "their health-giving resinous aroma," and of "little medicine, much milk, the tannin-impregnated wines." ". . . It is a subject for regret that a complaint, the recovery from which depends so much upon the patients' own wisdom and self-denial, should be more or less characteristic of an age when common sense and consistency are still at such a minimum. Thousands die before they are twenty-five out of inability to make sacrifices." See:

J. WEBER: *Illustrated Europe, Davos Guide Book,* 1880

7. Elizabeth Barrett Browning had her Greek books bound to look like novels, so that she might continue to read them despite her doctor's orders to the contrary.

CHAPTER XIV

1. However, an editorial in the *Lancet* of January, 1891, pointed out that the mortality of phthisis had decreased from 300 per 100,000 population in 1850 to 250 in 1860, and 220 in 1875. The decrease in mortality was traced by the author to improvement in hygienic conditions, draining of wet soil, better diets for the poor classes and control over the sale of the flesh of tuberculous animals.

The decline was not so obvious in other countries where industrialization had come later than in England. In Paris 12,314 of the 46,988 deaths registered in 1899 were attributed to tuberculosis. The disease accounted for three fifths of the mortality between the ages of twenty and forty.

2. Those who feel confident that everything is known of the factors responsible for the regression of tuberculosis in our communities

will do well to ponder over the case of several other diseases which, once very prevalent, have now all but vanished from Western Europe without benefit of scientific knowledge or empirical wisdom.

Leprosy is of particular interest for our story, because it is caused by a microorganism similar in many respects to the tubercle bacillus. The disease was once widespread in all parts of Europe and there are still today many millions of lepers throughout the world. Many theories have been formulated to account for its disappearance from sixteenth-century Europe — except from certain regions where it persisted until the twentieth century, particularly in Norway. Changes in weather, in nutrition, in living habits, and in sanitation have been regarded as responsible for rendering man more resistant to the leprosy bacillus, and for preventing the spread of infection. The segregation of lepers in leprosaria (of which there were many thousands in Europe during the Middle Ages) is often credited with the disappearance of the disease from Europe. The great epidemics of plague are assumed to have killed off the debilitated lepers crowded in the leprosaria. It is also stated that the repulsive character of the leprous lesions served as a sexual deterrent which resulted in the selective elimination of those endowed with natural susceptibility to the disease. Interesting as they are, all these hypotheses lack a convincing factual basis.

Unlike other diseases (for instance malaria and cholera) leprosy never became a public health problem in the Upper Mississippi Valley, despite the fact that it was introduced there by the Norwegian immigrants. Yet the living conditions among the latter were often most unsanitary, and their ways of life remained for several decades similar to those prevailing in their mother country where leprosy persisted much longer. It has not been possible to single out any factor, the presence or absence of which could explain the failure of leprosy to become established in the Mississippi Valley. See:

W. L. WASHBURN: *Leprosy among Scandinavian Settlers in the Upper Mississippi Valley*, 1864–1932, Bull. Hist. Med. 24, 1950, 123

Epidemiological facts have been presented during recent years to support the view that the increase in prevalence of tuberculosis has been one of the causes of the disappearance of leprosy. This hypothesis is based on the assumption (unproved) that the former disease can immunize against the latter. See:

R. CHAUSSINAUD: "Tuberculose et Lèpre. Maladies Antagoniques. Eviction de la Lèpre par la Tuberculose," *Intern. J. Leprosy* 16, 1948, 430

3. Recent epidemiological studies have contributed some further evidence for the view that it takes approximately one hundred years of tuberculosis epidemic in a fairly closed community to weed out the human strains most susceptible to the disease. The epidemiological history of tuberculosis in Mauritius, and also among the workers of the printing industry in England, can be cited as examples to the point. See:

MARGARET CARNS AND ALICE STEWART: "Pulmonary Tuberculosis in the Printing and Shoemaking Trades," *Brit. J. Soc. Med.*, 1951, 73

ALICE STEWART AND J. P. HUGHES: "Mass Radiography Findings in the Northamptonshire Boot and Shoe Industry," *Brit. Med. J.*, 1951, 899

4. The African Zebu cattle appear to be much more resistant to tuberculosis than are other breeds of cattle. Although they can become tuberculous under bad conditions of husbandry, their disease usually remains localized in the lungs and progresses very slowly.

5. In 1885, August Hirsch stated in his *Handbook:* "That phthisis propagates itself in many families from generation to generation is so much a matter of daily experience that the severest skeptic can hardly deny a hereditary element in the case." Nevertheless, it is difficult to prove the fact of familial susceptibility. For a modern treatment of the subject see:

R. R. PUFFER: *Familial Susceptibility to Tuberculosis.* Harvard University Press, Cambridge, 1944

6. This fact is illustrated by a recent report of the United States Navy Medical Corps, which shows that almost 90 per cent of the young recruits react negatively to the intradermal test with PPD.

7. Much of the literature on the rise and fall of tuberculosis among Indians and other races is discussed in McDougall's *Tuberculosis.* The introduction of tuberculosis in the Americas is also mentioned in:

P. M. ASHBURN: *The Ranks of Death.* Coward-McCann, New York, 1947

8. It appears that the American Indians are now reaching a state of greater resistance to tuberculosis. Although the rate of infection is still extremely high among them (most of the children becoming tuberculin-positive by the ages of ten to fifteen), only little more than 10 per cent of the total population show tuberculous lesions.

Of great interest is the fact that simple public health measures seem to have been effective in checking the spread of tuberculosis among the Indians. In Minnesota, there were 64 tuberculous deaths among the 12,500 Indians of the state in 1937; this number was reduced to 9 in 1949, although no program of vaccination had been instituted to supplement the usual procedures of tuberculosis control.

9. During the early part of the nineteenth century, the annual mortality of phthisis among the Negroes confined in the penitentiaries of Pennsylvania and Maryland reached the fantastic figure of 40 per 1000.

10. The pathological patterns of tuberculosis in different population groups provide further evidence of the fact that the natural history of the disease is influenced by the number of generations during which the group has been exposed to heavy infection. In the early phase of the epidemic, tuberculosis manifests itself as an acute generalized form, and finally becomes the chronic pulmonary tuberculosis which is now preponderant in most of the Western world.

An illustration of the same trend has been observed recently among the printer and shoemaker trades in England.

11. See for example:

"Tuberculosis in South Africa," *Tubercle* 31, 1950, 291

12. It was common to see extensive lesions predominantly of the caseous type. The course of the disease was often so rapid that there was no time for the production of cavities. When they formed, they were ill defined, with little or no evidence of fibrotic reaction. Healed lesions often became reactivated. Meningeal and generalized tuberculosis were extremely frequent even in adults.

13. See Chapter XI, Note 3.

CHAPTER XV

1. By contrast, an article in the London *National and Military Gazette* of 1851 affirmed that the wearing of mustaches was conducive to health by protecting the breathing apparatus, absorbing the cold of the air before it entered the nostrils, and thus acting as a preventative against consumption.

2. See:

S. A. K. Strahan: *Marriage and Disease, A Study of Heredity and the More Important Family Degenerations.* Appleton & Co., New York, 1892

3. General discussions of the effects of urbanization and industrialization on health are found in the following books and articles:

G. J. Drolet: "Epidemiology of Tuberculosis," in Goldberg's *Clinical Tuberculosis,* F. A. Davis, Philadelphia, 1946

JACK CECIL DRUMMOND AND WILBRAHAM: *The Englishman's Food.* Jonathan Cape, London, 1940
ALLAN K. KRAUSE: "Tuberculosis and Public Health," *Amer. Rev. Tub.* 18, 1928, 271
ALLAN K. KRAUSE: "Factors in the Pathogenesis of Tuberculosis," *Amer. Reb. Tub.* 18, 1928, 208
S. LEFF: *The Health of the People.* Victor Gollancz Ltd., London, 1950
MAX PINNER: "Epidemiological Trends of Tuberculosis," *Amer. Rev. Tub.* 42, 1940, 382
BERNHARD F. STERN: *Society and Medical Progress.* Princeton University Press, 1941
H. E. SIGERIST: *Civilization and Disease.* Cornell University Press, Ithaca, 1943
GEORGE WOLFF: "Tuberculosis Mortality and Industrialization (with Special Reference to the U. S.)," *Am. Rev. Tub.* 42, 1940, 214

4. "Like many of my contemporaries," wrote Thoreau in his *Journal,* "I had rarely for many years used animal food. . . . It appeared more beautiful to live low and fare hard."

CHAPTER XVI

1. See references listed in Chapter XV, Note 3.
2. For details concerning the genesis of the antituberculosis movement, see:

ROBERT G. PATERSON: *Antecedents of the National Tuberculosis Association.* N. T. A., New York, 1945.
RICHARD SHRYOCK: "The Historical Significance of the Tuberculosis Movement," in *Past and Present Trends in the Tuberculosis Movement,* National Tuberculosis Association, No. 886, 1942

3. In the Report of the sanitary commission of Massachusetts, published in 1850, Shattuck and others had already noted that consumption, "the dreadful disease, is a constant visitor in all parts of our Commonwealth," but creates little alarm because it is constantly present, whereas the occasional visit of cholera or some other epidemic disease stimulates precautionary measures.
4. See:

IAGO GALDSTON: "The Dynamics of Epidemiology in Relation to Epidemic Tuberculosis," *Amer. Rev. Tub.* 45, 1942, 609

5. See Chapter XII, Note 9.

6. Provisional figures recently compiled (August 1951) by the Statistical Service of the National Tuberculosis Association show that the death rate of tuberculosis in the United States was 22.2 per 100,000 population for 1950 (33,557 deaths) as against 26.1 for 1949 (38,870 deaths). The total number of new cases reported was 121,228 or 3.6 cases per death.

The twelve states with the lowest and highest tuberculosis death rates in 1950 were the following (death rates per 100,000 population in parentheses):

Lowest	*Highest*
Wyoming (3.8)	Arizona (68.2)
Utah (6.8)	District of Columbia (49.1)
Iowa (8.0)	New Mexico (35.7)
Nebraska (8.2)	Kentucky (34.1)
Idaho (9.4)	Maryland (33.8)
Kansas (10.0)	Tennessee (33.3)
Wisconsin (10.1)	Arkansas (31.3)
Minnesota (11.0)	Virginia (27.5)
New Hampshire (11.0)	Louisiana (27.5)
North Dakota (11.4)	Alabama (26.7)
Oregon (13.2)	Mississippi (25.6)
Washington (14.4)	New York (25.5)

It is obvious that mortality rates are the highest in all states with a large colored population. Most of the deaths in Arizona and New Mexico probably occur in the populations of Mexican and Indian origin, and among tuberculous patients who come to these states for treatment.

7. A recent analysis of the evolution of tuberculosis in the printing and shoe trades in England provides a striking example of the complex manner in which historical and social factors affect the course of the disease.

Prior to 1881, the first year for which statistical information is available, tuberculosis mortality was much higher in the printing industry than in the shoe industry, despite the fact that wages were better in the former than in the latter. But whereas tuberculosis decreased very rapidly among the printers after 1881, it did not among the shoemakers. A detailed study of the working conditions and of the recruitment of workers in the two industries during the past one hundred years seems to provide a satisfactory explanation for these peculiar epidemiological facts.

Since much of the work in printing and shoemaking does not demand strenuous labor, persons with some physical handicap, including those suffering from tuberculosis, often sought employment in these occupations. Thus, selective recruitment concentrated among printers and shoemakers individuals with chronic tuberculosis who served as foci for further spread of the disease in the two industries.

Industrialization began early in the printing trade and the centralization of workers in large factories facilitated the dissemination of bacilli. Also, as strong family traditions exist in the printing trade, a tuberculosis epidemic became established in the printers' community, causing at first great ravages, but later bringing about an increase in resistance in the families associated with printing, probably as a result of selection.

By contrast, industrialization did not begin until the 1880's in the shoe trade. And it appears that the tuberculosis mortality among shoemakers began to rise in comparison with that of other manual workers when they changed from working at home to working in factories, even though their wages improved with industrialization. Thus, the rise in relative tuberculosis death among shoemakers after 1881 corresponds to one of the usual effects of the first phases of industrialization, namely increase of exposure to infection while at work. Even now, the incidence of tuberculosis in the shoe trade is in direct relation to the size of factories and to the crowding in the workshops.

One of the practical results of this study has been to emphasize the importance of removing from immediate contact with their fellow workers the chronic carriers of bacilli, who constitute the most dangerous members of the community for the maintenance of infection. See:

ALICE STEWART AND J. P. HUGHES, *op. cit.* (Chapter XIV, Note 3)

MARGARET CAIRNS AND ALICE STEWART, *op. cit.* (Chapter XIV, Note 3)

8. By a macabre kind of arithmetic, it is possible to show that even in the United States, tuberculosis is still the cause of a greater loss of potential years of life and creative activity than are either heart diseases or cancer. See:

M. DEMPSEY. "Decline in Tuberculosis; the Death Rate Fails to Tell the Entire Story," *Amer. Rev. Tub.* 56, 1947, 157.

9.

H. R. EDWARDS AND G. J. DROLET: "The Implications of Changing Morbidity and Mortality Rates from Tuberculosis," *Amer. Rev. Tub.* 61, 1950, 39.

10. A striking change is also taking place in the age and sex distribution of tuberculosis. In our communities, the disease is found less and less among the young and more and more among the adult and old, particularly men. In Massachusetts, for instance, 60 per cent of all deaths from tuberculosis in 1949 were in men forty years old or more. Of the 3296 new cases reported in the male white population of New York City in 1949, 1892 were found among men over forty-five years of age.

As it is generally difficult to arrange for periodical medical examination of adults, those infected act as spreaders of bacilli for prolonged periods of time before they are detected. Moreover, the high proportion of adult tuberculous patients results in a large number of chronic cases whose welfare (and that of their families) constitutes a major economic problem. The number of chronic tuberculous patients taken care of by the Veterans Administration increases rapidly from year to year and will soon become one of its largest medical and financial burdens. See:

J. Barnwell: "Care of the Tuberculous Veteran, a Continuing Problem," *J. Amer. Med. Assoc.* 146, no. 15, 1951, 1372.

11. It is stated that a vast rehabilitation program of tuberculous patients is on foot in Russia. At the "Hammer and Sickle Works" in Kharkov, institutional medical treatment is combined with industrial occupation within the capabilities of the patient. Other facts concerning rehabilitation programs in different parts of the world are presented in McDougall's *Tuberculosis,* page 422, and in a survey, "The Rehabilitation and Care of the Tuberculous," published in *Tubercle,* January, 1942, pages 1 and 83.

One of the many interesting aspects of the Village Settlement program in England is the fact that there has not been a single death due to primary tuberculosis among the children living in the Settlement communities. And yet, there is at least one tuberculous member in each family, and infection can hardly be avoided. Here is telling evidence that tuberculosis can be conquered by enlightened medical policies and adequate living standards!

12. *J'aime mieux être homme à paradoxes qu'homme à préjugés.*

— Jean Jacques Rousseau

Index